An Update in Nephrology

Editors

JEFFREY M. TURNER
URSULA C. BREWSTER

MEDICAL CLINICS
OF NORTH AMERICA

www.medical.theclinics.com

Consulting Editor
JACK ENDE

July 2023 • Volume 107 • Number 4

ELSEVIER

1600 John F. Kennedy Boulevard • Suite 1800 • Philadelphia, Pennsylvania, 19103-2899

http://www.theclinics.com

MEDICAL CLINICS OF NORTH AMERICA Volume 107, Number 4
July 2023 ISSN 0025-7125, ISBN-13: 978-0-443-12983-4

Editor: Taylor Hayes
Developmental Editor: Malvika Shah

Medical Clinics of North America (ISSN 0025-7125) is published bimonthly by Elsevier Inc., 360 Park Avenue South, New York, NY 10010-1710. Months of publication are January, March, May, July, September, and November. Business and editorial offices: 1600 John F. Kennedy Boulevard, Suite 1800, Philadelphia, PA 19103-2899. Periodicals postage paid at New York, NY, and additional mailing offices. Subscription prices are USD $332.00 per year (US individuals), $786.00 per year (US institutions), $100.00 per year (US Students), $416.00 per year (Canadian individuals), $1023.00 per year (Canadian institutions), $200.00 per year for (foreign students), $100.00 per year for (Canadian students), $461.00 per year (foreign individuals), and $1023.00 per year (foreign institutions). To receive student/resident rate, orders must be accompanied by name of affiliated institution, date of term, and the signature of program/residency coordinator on institution letterhead. Orders will be billed at individual rate until proof of status is received. Foreign air speed delivery is included in all Clinics' subscription prices. All prices are subject to change without notice. **POSTMASTER:** Send address changes to *Medical Clinics of North America*, Elsevier Health Sciences Division, Subscription Customer Service, 3251 Riverport Lane, Maryland Heights, MO 63043. **Customer Service: Telephone: 1-800-654-2452** (U.S. and Canada); **1-314-447-8871** (outside U.S. and Canada). **Fax: 314-447-8029. E-mail: journalscustomerserviceusa@ elsevier.com** (for print support); **journalsonlinesupport-usa@elsevier.com** (for online support).

Reprints. For copies of 100 or more of articles in this publication, please contact the Commercial Reprints Department, Elsevier Inc., 360 Park Avenue South, New York, NY 10010-1710. Tel.: 212-633-3874; Fax: 212-633-3820; E-mail: reprints@elsevier.com.

Medical Clinics of North America is also published in Spanish by McGraw-Hill Interamericana Editores S. A., P.O. Box 5-237, 06500 Mexico, D.F., Mexico.

Medical Clinics of North America is covered in *MEDLINE/PubMed (Index Medicus), Current Contents, ASCA, Excerpta Medica, Science Citation Index,* and *ISI/BIOMED.*

PROGRAM OBJECTIVE

The goal of the *Medical Clinics of North America* is to keep practicing physicians up to date with current clinical practice by providing timely articles reviewing the state of the art in patient care.

TARGET AUDIENCE

All practicing physicians and other healthcare professionals.

LEARNING OBJECTIVES

Upon completion of this activity, participants will be able to:

1. Review various factors contributing to kidney disease.
2. Explain the importance of routine screening for early diagnosis and emerging new therapeutic interventions for kidney disease.
3. Discuss the pivotal role of the primary care physician in caring for and treating patients with kidney disease.

ACCREDITATION

The Elsevier Office of Continuing Medical Education (EOCME) is accredited by the Accreditation Council for Continuing Medical Education (ACCME) to provide continuing medical education for physicians.

The EOCME designates this journal-based CME activity for a maximum of 11 *AMA PRA Category 1 Credit*(s)™. Physicians should claim only the credit commensurate with the extent of their participation in the activity.

All other healthcare professionals requesting continuing education credit for this enduring material will be issued a certificate of participation.

DISCLOSURE OF CONFLICTS OF INTEREST

The EOCME assesses conflict of interest with its instructors, faculty, planners, and other individuals who are in a position to control the content of CME activities. All relevant conflicts of interest that are identified are thoroughly vetted by EOCME for fair balance, scientific objectivity, and patient care recommendations. EOCME is committed to providing its learners with CME activities that promote improvements or quality in healthcare and not a specific proprietary business or a commercial interest.

The planning committee, staff, authors, and editors listed below have identified no financial relationships or relationships to products or devices they or their spouse/life partner have with commercial interest related to the content of this CME activity:

Abinet M. Aklilu, MD, MPH; Ursula Brewster, MD; Mikhail Dmitriev, MD; Mary Dominguez, MD; Ladan Golestaneh, MD, MS; Maryam Gondal, MD; Sonali Gupta, MD; Kanza Haq, MD; Priyanka Jethwani, MBBS; Michelle Littlejohn; Wendy McCallum, MD, MS; Merlin Packiam; Dipal M. Patel, MD, PhD; Maria Jose Zabala Ramirez, MD; Arundati Rao, MBBS; Anushree Shirali, MD; Eva Stein, MD; Jeffrey M. Testani, MD, MTR; Jeffrey M. Turner, MD; Niloufarsadat Yarandi, MD

The planning committee, staff, authors, and editors listed below have identified financial relationships or relationships to products or devices they or their spouse/life partner have with commercial interest related to the content of this CME activity:

Justin Belcher, MD, PhD: Advisor: Mallinckrodt Pharmaceuticals

Koyal Jain, MD, MPH: Researcher: Visterra Inc., Kaneka Corporation

UNAPPROVED/OFF-LABEL USE DISCLOSURE

The EOCME requires CME faculty to disclose to the participants;

1. When products or procedures being discussed are off-label, unlabelled, experimental, and/or investigational (not US Food and Drug Administration [FDA] approved); and
2. Any limitations on the information presented, such as data that are preliminary or that represent ongoing research, interim analyses, and/or unsupported opinions. Faculty may discuss information about pharmaceutical agents that is outside of FDA-approved labelling. This information is intended solely for CME and is not intended to promote off-label use of these medications. If you have any questions, contact the medical affairs department of the manufacturer for the most recent prescribing information.

TO ENROLL

To enroll in the *Medical Clinics of North America* Continuing Medical Education program, call customer service at 1-800-654-2452 or sign up online at http://www.theclinics.com/home/cme. The CME program is available to subscribers for an additional annual fee of USD 282.00.

METHOD OF PARTICIPATION

In order to claim credit, participants must complete the following:

1. Complete enrolment as indicated above.
2. Read the activity.
3. Complete the CME Test and Evaluation. Participants must achieve a score of 70% on the test. All CME Tests and Evaluations must be completed online.

CME INQUIRIES/SPECIAL NEEDS

For all CME inquiries or special needs, please contact elsevierCME@elsevier.com.

MEDICAL CLINICS OF NORTH AMERICA

Contributors

CONSULTING EDITOR

JACK ENDE, MD, MACP
The Schaeffer Professor of Medicine, Perelman School of Medicine, University of Pennsylvania, Philadelphia, Pennsylvania

EDITORS

JEFFREY M. TURNER, MD
Associate Professor of Medicine, Section of Nephrology, Yale School of Medicine, New Haven, Connecticut

URSULA C. BREWSTER, MD
Professor of Medicine, Section of Nephrology, Yale School of Medicine, New Haven, Connecticut

AUTHORS

ABINET M. AKLILU, MD, MPH
Post doctoral fellow, Section of Nephrology, Department of Medicine, Yale School of Medicine, New Haven, Connecticut

JUSTIN M. BELCHER, MD, PhD
Associate Professor of Medicine, Section of Nephrology, Yale School of Medicine, VA Connecticut Healthcare System, VA Connecticut Healthcare, West Haven, Connecticut

URSULA C. BREWSTER, MD
Professor of Medicine, Section of Nephrology, Yale School of Medicine, New Haven, Connecticut

MIKHAIL DMITRIEV, MD
Resident physician, Department of Internal Medicine, Connecticut Institute for Communities (Danbury Hospital), Danbury, Connecticut

MARY DOMINGUEZ, MD
Assistant Professor, Department of Medicine, Division of Nephrology, Albert Einstein College of Medicine, Bronx, New York

LADAN GOLESTANEH, MD, MS
Professor, Department of Medicine, Division of Nephrology, Albert Einstein College of Medicine, Bronx, New York

MARYAM GONDAL, MD
Assistant Professor of Medicine, Department of Internal Medicine, Section of Nephrology, Yale School of Medicine, New Haven, Connecticut

SONALI GUPTA, MD
Assistant professor, Department of Medicine, Division of Nephrology, Albert Einstein College of Medicine, Bronx, New York

KANZA HAQ, MD
Division of Nephrology, Department of Internal Medicine, Johns Hopkins University, Baltimore, Maryland

KOYAL JAIN, MD, MPH
Associate Professor of Medicine, Division of Nephrology and Hypertension, Department of Medicine, UNC Kidney Center, The University of North Carolina at Chapel Hill, Chapel Hill, North Carolina

PRIYANKA JETHWANI, MBBS
Assistant Professor, Department of Surgery, The University of Tennessee Health Science Center, James D. Eason Transplant Institute, Methodist University Hospital, Memphis, Tennessee

WENDY MCCALLUM, MD, MS
Assistant professor of Medicine, Division of Nephrology, Tufts Medical Center, Boston, Massachusetts

DIPAL M. PATEL, MD, PhD
Assistant Professor of Medicine, Division of Nephrology, Department of Internal Medicine, Johns Hopkins University, Baltimore, Maryland

ARUNDATI RAO, MBBS
Nephrology Fellow, Yale School of Medicine, New Haven, Connecticut

ANUSHREE C. SHIRALI, MD
Associate Professor of Medicine, Section of Nephrology, Yale School of Medicine, New Haven, Connecticut

EVA J. STEIN, MD
Clinical Nephrology Fellow, Division of Nephrology and Hypertension, Department of Medicine, UNC Kidney Center, The University of North Carolina at Chapel Hill, Chapel Hill, North Carolina

JEFFREY M. TESTANI, MD, MTR
Associate Professor, Division of Cardiovascular Medicine, Yale School of Medicine, New Haven, Connecticut

JEFFREY M. TURNER, MD
Associate Professor of Medicine, Section of Nephrology, Yale School of Medicine, New Haven, Connecticut

NILOUFARSADAT YARANDI, MD
Assistant Professor of Medicine, Section of Nephrology, Yale School of Medicine, New Haven, Connecticut

MARIA JOSE ZABALA RAMIREZ, MD
Clinical Nephrology Fellow, Division of Nephrology and Hypertension, Department of Medicine, UNC Kidney Center, The University of North Carolina at Chapel Hill, Chapel Hill, North Carolina

Contents

Chronic kidney disease (CKD) is a silent progressive disease. It is diagnosed by assessing filtration and markers of kidney damage such as albuminuria. The diagnosis of CKD should include not only assessing the glomerular filtration rate (GFR) and albuminuria but also the cause. The CKD care plan should include documentation of the trajectory and prognosis. The use of a combination of serum cystatin C and creatinine concentration offers a more accurate estimation of GFR. Social determinants of health are important to address as part of the diagnosis because they contribute to CKD disparities.

Urinalysis is a widely used diagnostic tool to assist clinicians in determining the etiology of various acute or chronic pathologies. Primary care, general internal medicine, and family medicine clinicians should be adept at identifying indications for urinalyses, in addition to appropriately interpreting their results. In this article, we provide an overview of urinalysis for non-nephrologists.

Chronic kidney disease (CKD) is a progressive condition which is defined by decreased kidney function evidenced by a glomerular filtration rate (GFR) less than 60 mL/min per 1.73 m2 or markers of kidney damage, or both, for at least 3 months, regardless of the underlying cause. The 5 stages of CKD are based on the estimated GFR. Patients with CKD have significantly higher rates of morbidity, mortality, hospitalization, and health care utilization. Renal replacement therapy in the form of dialysis or kidney transplant is the life-sustaining treatment for patients with kidney failure. Predialysis education helps patients make informed decisions and opt for a modality conducive with their lifestyle/values. It has also been associated with improvement in measurable outcomes such as delayed initiation of dialysis, cardiovascular complications, and mortality.

Diabetes is a major public health challenge and diabetic kidney disease (DKD), a broader diagnostic term than diabetic nephropathy, is the leading cause of chronic kidney disease and end-stage kidney disease in the United States and worldwide. A better understanding of the underlying pathophysiological mechanisms of DKD, and recent clinical trials testing new therapeutic interventions, have shown promising results to curb this epidemic. Given the global health burden of DKD, it is extremely important to prioritize prevention, early recognition, referral, and aggressive management of DKD in the primary care setting.

Kidney transplantation remains the treatment of choice for eligible patients with end-stage kidney disease. The last few decades have seen an expansion in the transplant recipient pool with over 250,000 patients living with a kidney transplant today. Because of limited bandwidth for ongoing follow-up and management of chronic medical conditions, transplant centers are directing more and more patients back to their general nephrologists and primary care doctors for longitudinal care. As a result, it is becoming increasingly important for primary care physicians to have a nuanced understanding of medications, complications, and chronic medical problems unique to transplant recipients. This article reviews the role of the primary care office in helping streamline the pretransplant evaluation process and long-term posttransplant care.

Women pursue pregnancy with comorbidities such as hypertension and kidney disease, necessitating primary care physicians to remain up to date with current clinical practice. Hypertensive disorders of pregnancy pose risks to the pregnancy and to the woman in the short and long term. These risks and their management are detailed in this review. Normally, pregnancy is associated with hemodynamic and kidney-specific changes. Here the authors discuss these changes and review the impact and management of pregnancy-related acute kidney injury, chronic kidney disease, and dialysis in pregnant patients. Kidney transplant recipients may experience return of fertility and require counseling to improve outcomes.

Nephrotic syndrome (NS) is a key clinical entity for the internist to recognize and understand. A wide range of infectious, metabolic, malignant, and autoimmune processes drive nephrosis, leading to a syndrome defined by proteinuria, edema, and hypoalbuminemia. NS occurs due to increased permeability to proteins at the level of the glomerulus, which allows for passage of albumin and other proteins into the urine. Proteinuria leads to a cascade of clinical complications characterized by fluid accumulation, kidney inflammation, and dysregulation of coagulation and immunity. In this article, the authors review the clinically important etiologies of NS that should inform an initial clinical evaluation

Foreword
Early Detection of Kidney Disease

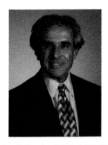

Jack Ende, MD, MACP
Consulting Editor

Kidney disease is often silent, but then it's not. There may be no warning signs or symptoms that a patient has lost substantial renal function until their disease is so advanced that life-altering renal replacement therapy must at least be considered.

In that sense, kidney disease is well-suited for screening and prevention. The criteria for medical conditions wherein early detection has a beneficial effect on outcomes should be well-known to us all. Simply put, those criteria include that the screening test is capable of detecting a high proportion of disease (ie, good sensitivity); that it is rarely positive in the absence of disease (ie, good specificity); that the cost of screening is reasonable, or at least not prohibitive; that the screening test should safe; and, of course, that it should lead to demonstrable and favorable impact on health outcomes.

These criteria are met when it comes to screening for chronic kidney disease. While many patients go on to advanced renal disease despite early detection, nihilism when it comes to preserving renal function is misplaced. Management of risk factors for kidney disease affects outcomes, while ignoring these risk factors can accelerate the onset of symptomatic disease. In addition, early detection of preclinical phases of kidney disease can allow the patient and physician to navigate a smoother transition when advanced stages are reached.

Hence, the importance of this issue of *Medical Clinics of North America*. The more we, as internal medicine and family physicians, know about kidney disease, and the more tuned in we are to early detection and prevention, the better the outcomes we can provide for our patients. This challenge, of course, has socioeconomic components having to do with access and equity. But for our patients in our offices and on our hospital services, we owe it to them to provide the best possible care.

Our guest editors, Drs Brewster and Turner, have assembled a highly qualified team of authors who provide up-to-date information on the panoply of nephrology conditions

Med Clin N Am 107 (2023) xiii–xiv
https://doi.org/10.1016/j.mcna.2023.04.003
0025-7125/23/© 2023 Published by Elsevier Inc.

that we encounter with our patients. This issue will be of great value as we all strive to detect, prevent, and treat kidney disease.

Jack Ende, MD, MACP
Perelman School of Medicine
University of Pennsylvania
Philadelphia, PA 19104, USA

E-mail address:
jack.ende@pennmedicine.upenn.edu

Preface

Kidney Health and Disease in 2023: An Update

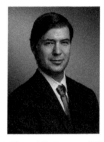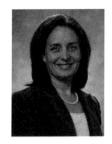

Jeffrey M. Turner, MD   Ursula C. Brewster, MD
Editors

Chronic kidney disease (CKD) remains a major health issue in the United States with up to 14% of the adult population having a low estimated glomerular filtration rate (GFR), albuminuria, or both based on recent data by the US Renal Data System, which is overseen by the National Institutes of Health. Diabetes and hypertension are the most common drivers of CKD and are increasing in our adult and pediatric population, as is obesity. These conditions are more common in patients from disadvantaged backgrounds, and in recent years, even our diagnostic methods have come under scrutiny for perpetuating that challenge. The management of patients with kidney diseases has changed rapidly in recent years. This has included the availability of multiple new medical therapies for CKD, new understanding about the pathogenesis of nephrotic syndromes, and a new focus on patients with oncologic diseases and kidney injury. In this issue, we have put together a collection of articles reviewing these key topics and others that are important and changing in the field of Nephrology today. We review how one diagnoses CKD in 2023 as the GFR equations have undergone some scrutiny of late and have been revised. We also include updates on cardiorenal syndrome, hepatorenal syndrome, and onconephrology, disorders that reflect the important relationship the kidneys have with other organ systems within the body. An in-depth review about kidney disease in pregnancy highlights the various pathologies that occur during gestation and the dangers these pose to both the developing fetus and the mother. Finally, core topics, such as diabetic kidney disease, hemodialysis, and secondary hypertension, are also covered. Our hope in this issue is to provide clinicians with valuable insights and understandings about caring for patients with kidney disease. This population is one of the most vulnerable within our health systems, reflected by the

Med Clin N Am 107 (2023) xv–xvi
https://doi.org/10.1016/j.mcna.2023.04.001
0025-7125/23/© 2023 Published by Elsevier Inc.

medical.theclinics.com

high rates of morbidity and mortality, expansive use of health care resources, and barriers to achieving improved quality of life. We hope you enjoy this issue.

Jeffrey M. Turner, MD
Section of Nephrology
Yale School of Medicine
330 Cedar Street
Boardman Building 114
New Haven, CT 06510, USA

Ursula C. Brewster, MD
Section of Nephrology
Yale School of Medicine
330 Cedar Street
Boardman Building 114
New Haven, CT 06510, USA

E-mail addresses:
jeffrey.turner@yale.edu (J.M. Turner)
ursula.brewster@yale.edu (U.C. Brewster)

Diagnosis of Chronic Kidney Disease and Assessing Glomerular Filtration Rate

Abinet M. Aklilu, MD, MPH

KEYWORDS

- CKD diagnosis • Kidney function • Chronic kidney disease • Estimating GFR
- Measuring GFR • Glomerular filtration rate • Monitoring GFR

KEY POINTS

- Chronic kidney disease diagnosis relies on the assessment of filtration function and evidence of kidney damage or dysfunction.
- Early diagnosis is essential to potentially reverse or halt the injury and slow the progression of kidney function decline.
- Identification of potentially modifiable risk factors for progression including chronic systemic diseases and nephrotoxic exposures and timely initiation of nephroprotective medications prevents the progression.
- Primary care providers have a critical role in early diagnosis of kidney dysfunction and prevention of its progression.

INTRODUCTION

Chronic kidney disease (CKD) is a progressive disease defined by international consensus guidelines as a glomerular filtration rate (GFR) of less than 60 mL/min per 1.73 m^2 body surface area or any evidence of kidney structural or functional abnormality present for more than 3 months.[1] Non-GFR evidence of kidney disease may include cystic disease, stone disease and sequelae, scarring or atrophy, renovascular disease, histologic or urinary findings of glomerular or interstitial disease, evidence of tubular dysfunction, and the presence of kidney transplant (**Fig. 1**). A chronicity criterion exists to distinguish CKD from acute kidney injury ($\leq$ 7 days) and disease ($\leq$ 3 months), emphasizing the importance of excluding reversible processes when making the diagnosis.[1,2] Although the chronicity criterion exists to distinguish acute from chronic kidney disease, it does not imply irreversibility or a missed opportunity for intervention. The kidneys, which are the major filtration, homeostasis, and metabolism apparatus of the body, often perform well in disease without obvious

Section of Nephrology, Department of Medicine, Yale school of Medicine, 60 Temple Street, Suite 6C, New Haven, CT 06510, USA
E-mail address: abinet.aklilu@yale.edu

Med Clin N Am 107 (2023) 641–658
https://doi.org/10.1016/j.mcna.2023.03.001
0025-7125/23/

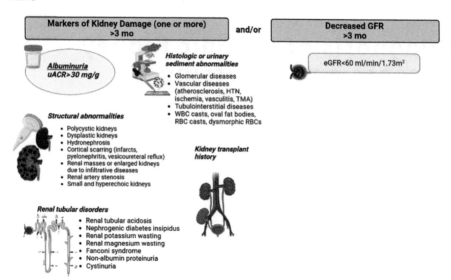

Fig. 1. Definitions of chronic kidney disease. CKD is defined as the presence of markers of kidney damage or decline in to a level less than 60 mL/min/1.73 m². Details of markers of kidney damage are shown according to the KDIGO 2012 guidelines.eGFR, estimated glomerular filtration rate; HTN, hypertension; RBC, red blood cell; TMA, thrombotic microangiopathy; uACR, urine albumin creatinine ratio; WBC, white blood cell.

evidence of dysfunction until severely impaired. However, although an apparently silent disease, CKD of even mild-to-moderate severity is an independent contributor to frailty as well as cardiovascular and all-cause mortality.[3–6] The causes of CKD are varied and can involve specific parts of the kidney with variable rates of progression. Regardless of the cause, the rate of kidney function decline may be slowed if diagnosed early and intervened on. The provider's primary mission in kidney care is therefore to identify risk factors and prevent the progression of CKD. Monitoring kidney function with regular screening, initiating nephroprotective medications early and modifying risk factors are the cornerstone of CKD management.

EPIDEMIOLOGY

CKD is an underestimated global public health issue affecting more than 10% of the world's population.[7] Its incidence, prevalence, and associated adverse outcomes continue to increase. More than 1 million deaths and additional 1.4 million cardiovascular deaths were attributable to CKD in 2017.[8] There were significant regional differences; notably in central America, CKD was the second leading cause of death, perhaps reflecting differences in causes and access to care.[7] In the US, according to the 2020 US Renal Data System (USRDS) report, an estimated 14% of the US population (~37 million people) lives with CKD.[9,10] CKD prevalence increases with age mirroring that of the major risk factors in the region—hypertension and diabetes. The prevalence of moderate-to-severe CKD was ~22% among those aged 65 years or older.[9] Despite the overwhelming burden of CKD, it is estimated that less than 10% of the US CKD population and 60% of those with severe CKD are aware of their kidney disease.[10,11]

CLASSIFICATION OF CHRONIC KIDNEY DISEASE

In an effort to standardize measurement and target prevention strategies, consensus definitions were put forth by the Kidney Disease | Improving Global Outcomes (KDIGO) consortium.[12] The KDIGO stratifies CKD into 5 GFR categories, where stage 1 represents normal kidney function and stage 5 signifies the most advanced kidney disease heralding the ensuing need for kidney replacement therapy (KRT)[12] (**Fig. 2**). The staging includes GFR, urinary albumin concentration and a chronicity criterion. An estimated GFR (eGFR) less than 60 mL/min/1.73 m^2 and/or a urinary albumin-to-creatinine ratio (uACR) > 30 mg/g for greater than 3 months signifies CKD. The guideline-recommended classification system for documentation and monitoring and prognostication is the CGA classification system, which incorporates the cause (C), GFR (G), and degree of albuminuria (A). Kidney disease can also be classified based on the structure involved[1] (**Table 1**).

RATIONALE FOR EARLY DIAGNOSIS

The benefit of early diagnosis of CKD is multifold. Late diagnosis and delayed nephrology referrals have been associated with higher mortality, poor control of CKD complications, lower utilization of optimal modalities and late evaluation for vascular access and kidney transplant.[13,14] Major benefits of CKD diagnosis therefore include early risk factor modification, psychosocial preparedness, timely palliative care evaluation and KRT-planning including discussion of home modalities, vascular access, transplant evaluation, and identification and management of CKD-related complications such as metabolic acidosis, anemia, and mineral bone disease.

CKD is associated with adverse cardiovascular outcomes even at the earliest stages.[5,15] Furthermore, drugs that have nephroprotective benefits have shown cardiovascular benefits.[16–19] During the past decade, there has been accelerated growth in CKD therapy research, a major progress since the discovery of renin-angiotensin-system inhibitors (RASis). RASis work by mitigating glomerular hypertension via glomerular afterload reduction lowering albuminuria, a well-known risk factor for the

Prognosis of CKD by GFR and Albuminuria Categories: KDIGO 2012			Persistent Albuminuria Categories		
			A1	A2	A3
			Normal to mildly increased	Moderately increased	Severely increased
			ACR < 30 mg/g	ACR 30-299 mg/g	ACR ≥ 300 mg/g
GFR Categories (ml/min/1.73m²) Description and Range	G1	Normal or High ≥90			
	G2	Mildly Decreased 60-90			
	G3a	Mildly to Moderately Decreased 45-59			
	G3b	Moderately to Severely Decreased 30-44			
	G4	Severely Decreased 15-29			
	G5	Kidney Failure <15			

Fig. 2. KDIGO classifications of CKD and associated prognosis. ACR, albumin creatinine ratio; CKD, chronic kidney disease; GFR, glomerular filtration rate. The darker the shade of blue the poorer the prognosis. (*Adapted from* Chapter 1: Definition and classification of CKD. Kidney Int Suppl (2011). 2013 Jan;3(1):19-62. https://doi.org/10.1038/kisup.2012.64. PMID: 25018975; PMCID: PMC4089693.)

Table 1
Classifications of kidney dysfunction, injury patterns, and examples of causes

Type of Kidney Dysfunction	Pattern of Injury	Causes	
		Predisposing Diseases	Predisposing Drugs
Glomerular disease	Minimal change disease	Malignancies (hematologic more often)	NSAIDs (most common)
		Infections (syphilis, TB, HIV)	Selective COX-2 inhibitors, bisphosphonates, lithium, immune checkpoint inhibitors
		Autoimmune diseases	
	Membranous nephropathy	Solid organ cancer, autoimmune—Lupus	NSAIDs
		Infection—HBV	Penicillamine, parenteral gold, and mercurial salts
	FSGS	APOL-1 nephropathy, obesity, HTN, low nephron endowment (surgical/congenital atrophic or solitary kidney, premature birth/low birthweight), chronic reflux, healed inflammatory GN, Infections (HIV, EBV, CMV, parvovirus B19)	NSAIDs, interferon, pamidronate, heroin, anabolic steroids
	Membrano-proliferative GN	Cirrhosis—IgAN, Infections—HBV, HCV	Heroin, alpha-interferon
		Complement-mediated GN	
		TMA, transplant glomerulopathy	
		Plasma cell dyscrasias/MGRS	
		Autoimmune—most commonly SLE	
	Nodular glomerulosclerosis	Diabetes, amyloidosis, monoclonal immunoglobulin deposition disease	Tobacco

Tubulointerstitial diseases	Tubulointerstitial abnormalities			
	Interstitial nephritis		Infiltrative disease (leukemia, lymphoma)	NSAIDs, antibiotics, immune checkpoint inhibitors,
			Granulomatous disease, IgG4 disease, TINU	Lead, aristolochic acid
			Infections (eg, EBV, CMV, granuloma forming—TB, parasites, spirochetes)	
	Cystic disease		Acquired from CKD	Lithium
			Inherited (eg, ADPKD, ADTKD, medullary nephrocalcinosis, tuberous sclerosis complex, VHL, nephronophthisis)	
	Stone disease/ nephrocalcinosis		Primary hyperoxaluria, inherited tubulopathies	Topiramate, heavy oxalate intake (excessive vitamin C), vitamin D therapy, fat malabsorption (orlistat)
			RTA type I, granulomatous disease	
			Medullary sponge kidney	
			Chronic hypokalemia	
	Electrolyte disturbances	Hypokalemia and hypomagnesemia	Inherited tubulopathies (eg, Bartter, Gitelman)	PPIs, diuretics, cisplatin, EGFR inhibitors
		Hyponatremia	SIADH—cancer, cerebral lesion	NSAIDs, thiazides, psychotropics (SSRI/SNRI), cisplatin, MTX, ifosfamide, MDMA (ecstasy), linezolid, opiates, interferon, desmopressin
		DI	Hereditary, hypercalcemia, hypokalemia, urinary tract obstruction, sickle cell trait/disease	Lithium, ifosfamide, V2 receptor antagonist, foscarnet, cidofovir, amphotericin B, demeclocycline, orlistat
		RTA	Granulomatous/autoimmune disease, diabetes, obstruction, advanced CKD, sickle cell disease, plasma cell dyscrasia	NSAIDs, topiramate, cisplatin, gentamycin, ifosfamide, tenofovir disoproxil fumarate
		Hypercalcemia	Hyperparathyroidism, granulomatous dz, MM, hyperthyroidism	Lithium, vitamin D, calcium, thiazide

(continued on next page)

Table 1
(continued)

Type of Kidney Dysfunction	Pattern of Injury	Causes	
		Predisposing Diseases	Predisposing Drugs
Vascular	Ischemic nephropathy	Hypercalcemia	CNI (tacrolimus, cyclosporin)
	• Vasospasm induced	Hypertension/renovascular disease/ FMD	Cocaine
	• Renovascular disease	Atheroembolic disease	
		TMA, vasculitis (eg, ANCA-associated vasculitis)	

Abbreviations: ADPKD, autosomal dominant polycystic kidney disease; ADTKD, autosomal dominant tubulointerstitial kidney disease; ANCA, antineutrophil cytoplasmic antibodies; CKD, chronic kidney disease; CMV, cytomegalovirus; CNI, calcineurin inhibitor; DI, diabetic insipidus; EBV, Epstein-Barr virus; FMD, fibromuscular dysplasia; FSGS, focal segmental glomerulosclerosis; HBV, hepatitis B virus; HCV, hepatitis C virus; MM, multiple myeloma; MTX, methotrexate; NSAIDs, nonsteroidal anti-inflammatory drugs; PPI, proton pump inhibitor; RTA, renal tubular acidosis; SIADH, syndrome of inappropriate antidiuretic hormone; SLE, systemic lupus erythematosus; TB, tuberculosis; TINU, tubulointerstitial nephritis and uveitis; TMA, thrombotic microangiopathy; V2 receptor, vasopressin-2 receptor; VHL, von-Hippel Lindau.

CKD progression.[20,21] Two additional classes of drugs have shown consistent nephroprotective effects.[17,18,22,23] The sodium-glucose cotransporter-2 inhibitors are proven to slow the progression of kidney disease and cardiovascular outcomes in adults with and without diabetes with wide range of GFR.[16–18] Finerenone, a first-in-class nonsteroidal mineralocorticoid receptor antagonist, has also shown reduction in CKD progression and gained FDA approval for its antifibrotic effects in diabetes-associated CKD as well as heart failure.[19,22,24] This progress is worth emphasis as the most important risk factor contributing to the burden of CKD particularly in the North American region is diabetes. Among 785,883 US persons living with end-stage kidney disease (ESKD) in 2018, the disease was attributed to diabetes or hypertension in 65%, with diabetes identified as the primary cause in ~40%.[9,10] According to the 2022 USRDS report, 60% of the ESKD population has diabetes.[25] With 1 out of 5 people in the US believed to have diabetes, the burden of diabetic CKD is expected to increase further.[10]

Etiologies of Chronic Kidney Disease and Risk Factors for Progression

CKD develops from various causes, which may be systemic or primary kidney in nature. Acute or subacute insults that are prolonged or repeated often result in chronic changes especially when the baseline reserve is poor. Acute insults may include ischemic or nephrotoxin-induced acute tubular injury, urinary tract obstruction, and acute glomerulonephritis. Chronic causes are often from chronic conditions such as diabetes and hypertension, inherited glomerular or tubulointerstitial diseases and chronic cumulative exposure to nephrotoxins. Identifying the cause is a key part of the diagnosis of CKD. Once acute causes of kidney dysfunction are excluded, identifying the cause further aids in targeted prognostication and risk factor reduction including glycemic and blood pressure control, avoidance of nephrotoxins, and initiation of nephroprotective medications. Even when the duration of dysfunction is prolonged, the progression may be halted or slowed if modifiable risk factors are identified.

Risk factors for CKD progression: The minimum change in GFR that signifies rapid progression is 25% or 5 mL/min/1.73 m^2/y.[1,26] Faster 1-year progression of 25% or greater decline in has been associated with worse outcomes including ESKD and all-cause mortality.[12,27–30] Factors that influence the likelihood and rate of CKD progression include baseline GFR; the degree of albuminuria; the cause of kidney disease; ongoing exposure to nephrotoxic agents; obesity; hypertension; age; race/ethnicity; socioeconomic status; and laboratory parameters such as hemoglobin, albumin, calcium, phosphate, and bicarbonate.[17]

Risk estimation: In an effort to encourage early prevention strategies at the primary care level, CKD progression risk equations have been explored.[31] The kidney failure risk equation (KFRE) has been validated in multiple countries.[32–36] The KFRE allows estimation of 2-year and 5-year progression risk in adults with an eGFR of less than 60 mL/min/1.73 m.[2,32] A site that provides information for patients, BP goals and degree of risk reduction with BP control alone and with the initiation of specific nephroprotective drug classes is available for use at the primary health care level: https://kidneyfailurerisk.com/.

DIAGNOSIS OF CHRONIC KIDNEY DISEASE

The diagnosis of CKD includes assessing the stage, ascertaining the cause, and examining the rate of disease progression. Assessment of kidney function starts with estimating the GFR and assessing the degree of albuminuria. The KDIGO categories are presented in **Fig. 2** where stage G1A1 represents GFR greater than 90 mL/min/1.73 m^2 and uACR less than 30 mg/g. An initial recognition of GFR decline should be investigated as a possible acute kidney injury. As such, potential reversible causes must be explored to ensure early diagnosis to prevent scarring. Besides a detailed history and physical examination, a basic evaluation of kidney dysfunction includes urine analysis, quantification of proteinuria and kidney ultrasound with postvoid residual assessment if symptoms indicate. A prevention-focused diagnostic guide for CKD is shown (**Fig. 3**).

The history: History should include a comprehensive review of comorbidities including other organ dysfunction; personal and family history of kidney disease; systemic or genitourinary symptoms including rheumatologic symptoms, hematuria, or frothy urine; symptoms of bladder outlet obstruction (ie, poor flow, incomplete bladder emptying, frequency, urgency, hesitancy, nocturia); symptoms of volume overload; a complete review of prescribed, over-the-counter and herbal drugs; and family history. Medications such as proton pump inhibitors (PPIs), antimicrobials, nonsteroidal anti-inflammatory drugs (NSAIDs), immunosuppressants, and certain oncotherapeutic agents may cause interstitial nephritis or glomerulonephritis of varying trajectory. It is important to review prescribed and over-the-counter drugs at every visit and discontinue those that are not necessary. History should also include the assessment of social determinants of health, which must be considered when devising a management strategy.[37]

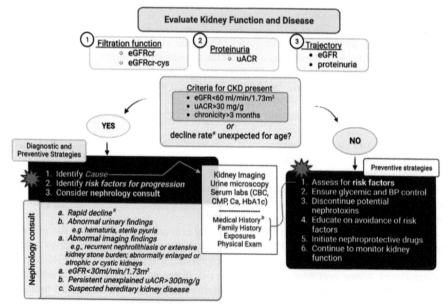

Fig. 3. Prevention-focused evaluation of chronic kidney disease. The diagnosis of CKD incorporates evaluation of filtration, presence of kidney damage and the rate of progression as well as the cause of the dysfunction. BP, blood pressure; Ca, calcium; CMP, comprehensive metabolic panel; eGFR, estimated glomerular filtration rate; eGFRcr, estimated glomerular filtration rate using creatinine; eGFRcr-cys, estimated glomerular filtration rate using creatinine and cystatin; HbA1c, hemoglobin A1c; uACR, urine albumin-to-creatinine ratio. [a]Significant decline rate is defined as annual decline by more than 5 mL/min/1.73 m^2 or by 25% from baseline. [b]Medical history includes personal history of systemic and kidney diseases that are risk factors for CKD and its progression. Figure created with Biorender.

Physical examination: Examination of the patient with CKD should include vital signs assessment, comprehensive assessment of volume status including orthostatic blood pressure and heart rate, evaluation for signs of volume overload, signs of heart and liver failure, and microvascular complications of diabetes and hypertension. Additionally, frailty is a potentially modifiable complication that should be assessed.[38] Abnormal findings should be investigated with further tests and interventions accordingly.

Laboratory Investigation

Serum studies: A comprehensive metabolic panel and complete blood count (CBC) with differential should be part of the initial workup of CKD. Laboratory parameters could reveal potential causes as well as CKD-related complications. For example, hypercalcemia may suggest primary hyperparathyroidism, or exogenous or endogenous causes (eg, vitamin D intoxication, sarcoidosis, paraneoplastic, or dysproteinemia). CBC may reveal evidence of systemic diseases such as hematologic malignancies or complications of advanced kidney disease such as anemia. Hypoalbuminemia may be an evidence of nephrotic syndrome.

Urine studies: Urine studies including urinalysis with microscopy should be obtained as the initial workup of kidney dysfunction. New onset dipstick proteinuria with or without GFR decline should be investigated with uACR as albuminuria is a major risk factor for CKD progression.[20,21] Proteinuria more than 3 g/d or uACR greater than 2200 mg/g signifies nephrotic range proteinuria and requires urgent nephrology referral for glomerulonephritis evaluation.[1] Urinalysis may also reveal microscopic hematuria, where greater than 20 RBCs per high-power-field (HPF) is considered significant.[26] Hematuria may develop from nephrolithiasis, cyst rupture, or a lesion along the urinary tract but may also signify inflammatory glomerulonephritis. Glomerular and lower urinary tract hematuria are differentiated from each other by the presence of dysmorphic red blood cells (RBCs) and RBC casts on urine microscopy in the former. The presence of sterile pyuria and/or white blood cell casts may indicate urinary tract inflammation or tubulointerstitial nephritis, which is often drug-associated. Urine microscopy may also show crystals suggestive of an underlying stone disease and should lead to detailed dietary and supplement exposure evaluation. Kidney dysfunction may also be the earliest sign of a hematologic malignancy presenting in the form of infiltrative disease or monoclonal gammopathy of renal significance (MGRS).[39] Patients with proteinuria with or without albuminuria particularly in the setting of anemia and hypercalcemia warrant an investigation into plasma cell dyscrasias such as multiple myeloma or MGRS. A dedicated discussion of urinalysis is provided in Chapter 2.

Imaging studies: Imaging studies such as ultrasound of the kidney and bladder help exclude obstruction and assess chronicity of kidney dysfunction. Ultrasound may reveal obstructive or nonobstructive stone, renal masses and cysts of varying sizes, and anatomic abnormalities that could be congenital or acquired such as atrophic kidney from renovascular disease and cortical abnormalities following infections, infarcts, or trauma. Ultrasound also serves as a prognostic tool by allowing the assessment of chronicity based on the kidney length, preservation of cortical thickness, and cortical echogenicity.[40,41] In addition, if available, ultrasound can assist in the evaluation of volume status at the point-of-care. Point-of-care ultrasound can be an invaluable tool and an extension to the physical examination particularly in the management of patients with poorly compensated liver disease and heart failure.[42]

Nephrologist evaluation: A persistent acute kidney injury, rapid progression of CKD (ie, an annual decline in greater than 25% or 5 mL/min/1.73 m^2), less than 30 mL/min/1.73 m,[2] persistent unexplained proteinuria (uACR $\geq$300 mg/g), RBC casts or persistent hematuria of greater than 20 RBCs/HPF, recurrent nephrolithiasis, and hereditary kidney disease warrant a nephrologist consultation.[1,12] Rapid sustained decline should raise concern for a rapidly progressive glomerulonephritis, which warrants an urgent kidney biopsy and therapy initiation accordingly. Generally, suspicion for an intrinsic inflammatory kidney disease such as glomerulonephritis or interstitial nephritis warrants a more urgent nephrologist evaluation for timely diagnosis and therapy initiation. Non- indications for a nephrologist referral also include poorly controlled hypertension, structural abnormalities including extensive kidney stones, higher number of kidney cysts than expected for age, and persistent electrolyte abnormalities. Late nephrology referrals have been associated with higher mortality, poor control of CKD complications such as anemia, lower utilization of home dialysis modalities, and late referral for vascular access and kidney transplant.[13,14] Risk, rather than GFR cutoff-based nephrology referral, may reduce CKD progression and mitigate such outcomes.[43]

Genetic screening: Genetic screening may aid in the diagnosis and prognostication of kidney dysfunction and may be pursued in consultation with a nephrologist. Genetic screening may particularly reveal a glomerular disease of variable course and help initiate treatment early in some cases and avoid unnecessary treatments in others. The 2022 KDIGO conclusions on genetics in CKD highlight the following benefits: early initiation of general nephroprotective therapies, initiation of targeted therapies, avoidance of potentially harmful or futile drugs, and surveillance for recurrence of disease after kidney transplantation.[44]

ASSESSING GLOMERULAR FILTRATION RATE

Assessment of GFR is a key component of CKD diagnosis. As a noninvasive study, it has been the primary method of defining and stratifying CKD (see **Fig. 2**). In steady states, GFR is routinely estimated using endogenous markers. GFR-estimating formulae must not be used to assess kidney function in nonsteady states such as acute kidney injury or disease.

Definition

GFR is defined as the cumulative amount of plasma filtered by all nephrons per unit time. The average kidneys receive a net of 20% to 25% of the total cardiac output per minute, filtering on average 180 L of plasma volume a day. Although this is the amount that enters Bowman space, only about 1.5 L urine output is produced on average because of the highly specialized reabsorption function of the kidney tubules. The kidneys are also responsible for regulating fluid and electrolyte balance, blood pressure, water and thirst, drug metabolism and excretion, gluconeogenesis, bone mineral metabolism and erythropoiesis, most of which they can resiliently perform until severely impaired.[45] Therefore, it should be noted that filtration is only one component of kidney function. Normal GFR in adults is reported as 100 to 130 mL/min/1.73 m^2 although this is likely lower in older adults.

Glomerular Filtration Rate Evaluation and Its Progress

GFR has been used as a measure of kidney function for nearly a century.[46–49] GFR can be measured using the urinary or plasma clearance of intravenously infused exogenous markers or estimated using endogenous markers. The ideal filtration marker is one with low protein binding and not secreted, metabolized, or reabsorbed by the kidney tubules. The gold standard is inulin, a fructose polysaccharide that is freely filtered and excreted without reabsorption or secretion.[50] Hence, $GFR = C_{inulin} = \frac{U_{inulin}}{P_{inulin}} \times V,$

where C_{inulin} = clearance of inulin in milliliters per minute, U_{inulin} = urine concentration of inulin in milligrams per milliliter, P_{inulin} = plasma concentration of inulin milligrams per milliliter, and V = urine flow rate. However, this is impractical and not routinely done in the clinical setting. In clinical practice, GFR is estimated using the more practical endogenous markers, most commonly serum creatinine, which is a product of creatine breakdown in skeletal muscle.

The innovation of endogenous marker-based equations for GFR estimation has made significant contribution to the advancement of kidney care from epidemiologic assessments that affect policy change and drive further research to large-scale assessments of kidney outcomes in response to therapeutics.[12,16–18] Equations for the estimation of kidney function have existed for more than half-a-century.[51] Although the biomarker used to estimate GFR has not changed, progress has been achieved in at least two major areas: standardization of biomarker assays and estimating equations. Standardized assays with creatinine concentrations calibrated to be traceable to the gold-standard isotope dilution mass spectrometry (IDMS) method have been widely adopted to reduce bias.[52] Moreover, GFR estimation has evolved during the past 2 decades with an increasing emphasis on broadening the diversity of the derivation cohorts to improve generalizability.[50,53] The Cockcroft-Gault equation of 1976, the first widely adopted in clinical practice, was derived using a cohort of 249 Caucasian male hospitalized veterans aged 18 to 92 and included age and weight.[51] Because it became commonly used in the pharmacokinetic assessment of drugs developed during the following decades, dosing recommendations of numerous drugs use clearance cutoffs based on this equation.[54] The next widely adopted equation was the Modified Diet in Renal Disease (MDRD) equation (published in 1999 and revised with IDMS-standardized assay in 2006), which included a more diverse cohort (n = 1628 adults) with the inclusion of women (40%) and African Americans (12%).[55] A 4-variable equation containing serum creatinine, age, sex, and race was found to have the best approximation to GFR measured using urinary clearance of 125-I-iothalamate.[55] It had better accuracy than the Cockcroft-Gault or creatinine clearance measurement but has greater bias in eGFR greater than 60 mL/min/1.73 m^2 because it was developed in a CKD cohort. The 2009 CKD epidemiology (CKD-EPI) equations were developed to improve on the imprecision of the MDRD.[56] The CKD-EPI pooled data from 10 unique study cohorts for development and 16 other studies for validation and found a regression model containing serum creatinine, age, sex, and race to best approximate measured GFR. At the time, cystatin C, a 13-kDa molecule produced by all nucleated cells unaffected by body size or dietary intake, was being studied as a more accurate alternative or addition to creatinine.[57,58] CKD-EPI cystatin C and combined creatinine-cystatin C-based equations were developed in 2012.[57] Although cystatin C-based equation did not require race, it did not perform better than the creatinine-based equation suggesting effects of non-GFR determinants. However, the combined creatinine-cystatin C equation performed better than those based on creatinine or cystatin C alone and was subsequently included in the 2012 KDIGO CKD guidelines.[12,57] Efforts to encourage widespread use of cystatin C are ongoing but practicality is still limited due to cost.

Although there was some improvement in diversity in the CKD-EPI datasets with the inclusion of entirely African American (African American Study of Kidney Disease and Hypertension) and Pima Indian (Diabetic Renal Disease Study) cohorts, the generalizability of the equation was questioned. More recently, broader racial justice movements that questioned the use of race as a biological explanation led to reevaluation by a national multidisciplinary Task Force and development of a new race-free equation.[59,60] A new creatinine and cystatin C-based equation was developed in 2021 using data pooled from multiple study cohorts refit with the same methods as in the 2012 study without race as an explanatory variable.[60] Closer to 90% of the eGFR were within 30% of corresponding measured-GFR making these equations more accurate than previous equations. Widespread adoption of the new equation is taking place nationally along with promotion of easier access to cystatin C and nationwide initiatives for more accurate biomarker research.

Pitfalls of eGFR and Chronic Kidney Disease Classifications

1. Although eGFR helps estimate, risk-stratify and monitor patients' kidney function, it is limited by non-GFR determinants of the biomarker used. In addition to GFR, the generation, tubular secretion, tubular reabsorption, and extrarenal excretion also affect the plasma concentration of an endogenous filtration marker (**Fig. 4**).[61] The variable inclusion of populations with different stages of CKD, smoking, obesity, work, and dietary intake contribute to inaccuracies compared with measured GFR as the marker used is sensitive to these factors. Creatinine concentration can be influenced by factors that alter its tubular secretion such as the drugs trimethoprim and cimetidine and possibly genetics and factors that affect its generation such as diet, genetics, edematous states, and extremes of body weight and muscle mass.[53] In comparison, cystatin C is freely filtered, not secreted in the proximal convoluted tubules and is produced by all nucleated cells at a constant rate although with some influence by corticosteroids and possibly diabetes and adiposity.[50] Although cost limits its widespread use at this time, cystatin C should be used when a more accurate GFR assessment is needed such as for medication dosing or referral considerations.[59]

2. GFR is not a comprehensive measure of kidney function. It is insensitive to detecting slowly progressive interstitial disease and proteinuric glomerular disease where filtration may be preserved until there is a significant nephron loss. This makes urine

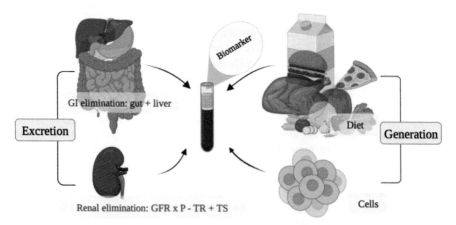

Fig. 4. Determinants of serum concentrations of endogenous filtration markers. The plasma concentration of an endogenous marker is a net balance of its generation (from diet and cellular production) and its elimination via the gastrointestinal system and urinary excretion, the latter a balance between the filtered load (GFR × P) and tubular secretion and tubular reabsorption. GFR, glomerular filtration rate; GI, gastrointestinal; P, plasma level; TR, tubular reabsorption; TS, tubular secretion. Created using Biorender. (Adapted with minor modification from *Stevens and Levey et al* with permission.[79])

analysis an important complement to GFR measurement. Albuminuria, in particular, has been associated with CKD progression[62,63] while the reduction of protein-uria has been shown to slow CKD progression.[64]

3. Normal aging is associated with a physiologic, nonpathologic GFR decline of about 4.9 mL/min/1.73 m^2 per decade.[61] All current equations are known to overestimate measured GFR in older adults. The CKD classification may overdiagnose mild and moderate CKD in older age individuals who experience GFR decline due to age-related nephron loss or glomerulosclerosis. Special attention must be given to the eGFR trajectory in such settings.

4. Using a single cutoff for CKD across all ages and discounting all greater than 60 mL/min/1.73 m^2 as normal in the CKD classification may also lead to underdi-agnosis or cause a delay in diagnosis in younger individuals.[65] Therefore, it is important to monitor the biomarker and trend and treat evidence of kidney damage early regardless of eGFR.

Special Considerations: Social Determinants of Health

The US Department of Health and Human Services defines social determinants of health (SDoH) as circumstances that people are born into, live, grow, and age that influence their health, which can be grouped into 5 domains: economic stability; education access and quality; neighborhood and built environment; social and community context; and health-care access and quality.[37,66] These include access to nutritious foods and physical activity, language and literacy, and cumulative exposure to overwhelming stressors such as discrimination, food insecurity and concerns for safety, often termed allostatic load.[67] Socioeconomic factors such as income, homelessness, food insecurity, and education attainment in particular have been shown to influence the development and progression of CKD.[68–70]

Special attention must also be paid to immigrant communities where the risk factors and age distributions of CKD and barriers to care may be different. CKD of unknown cause (CKDu), also known as Chronic Interstitial Nephritis of Agricultural Communities or Meso-American Nephropathy is a progressive interstitial kidney disease increasingly being reported in rural agricultural communities and should be considered in patients immigrating from endemic areas.[71,72] CKD is now the second leading cause of death in Central America and fifth in Andean Latin America possibly secondary to this unexplained epidemic.[7] Climate change and environmental toxins such as fertilizers and pesticides have been postulated but no consistent cause has been identified.[71] Furthermore, separate from the contributions of systemic socioeconomic and access-based differences, having 2 APOL1 risk alleles was recognized as a CKD progression accelerant in people of recent African descent.[73,74] These variants are thought to have developed 10,000 years ago to confer resistance to the deadly trypanosomiasis.[74] An estimated 13% of the African American population and 5% to 50% of the sub-Saharan population (Southern, Western, Central and pockets of East Africa) is thought to have 2 high-risk alleles, although not all with 2 risk alleles develop CKD suggesting the necessity of a trigger (second hit).[74,75] Having 2 risk alleles has been associated with collapsing-type focal segmental glomerulosclerosis, HIV-associated nephropathy, hypertension-attributed ESKD, lupus with severe kidney features, sickle cell nephropathy, nondiabetic CKD, and now COVID-19 infection.[76–78]

SDoH, including barriers to care, must therefore be considered especially in high-risk populations undergoing kidney function evaluation. Documenting and tackling SDoH and focusing on prevention may reduce the burden of advanced CKD and its complications on a broader scale.

SUMMARY

The assessment of GFR is only one component in the diagnosis of CKD. The diagnosis of CKD must also include quantifying albuminuria and identifying the cause and assessing rate of progression. There is currently no measure of kidney function that is both highly accurate and efficient to implement widely in clinical practice. Review of medications is necessary with focus on elimination or substitution of nephrotoxins wherever possible. Psychosocial factors including social determinants of health are important to address as part of the diagnosis and monitoring of CKD because they contribute to health disparities and outcomes by presenting major barrier to effective treatment strategies.

CLINICS CARE POINTS

- CKD is characterized according to the CGA criteria: the cause, GFR less than 60 mL/min/1.73 m^2 and/or albuminuria 30 mg/day or greater, and/or structural abnormalities present for greater than 3 months.

- In the diagnosis of CKD, the rate of kidney disease progression must be considered, all reversible causes excluded, and risk factors for the progression identified because targeting modifiable risk factors early can delay its progression.

- Because measurement of GFR is impractical for routine clinical use, GFR is estimated using endogenous filtration markers, which may be influenced by non-GFR determinants.

- Using a combination of creatinine and cystatin C offers a better estimation of kidney function in states that affect creatinine generation such as extremes of muscle mass.

DISCLOSURE

The author has nothing to disclose.

REFERENCES

1. Kidney Disease Improving Global Outcomes (KDIGO). Chapter 1: Definition and classification of CKD. Kidney Int Suppl 2013;3(1):19–62.
2. On behalf of the Acute Disease Quality Initiative Workgroup 16, Chawla LS, Bellomo R, et al. Acute kidney disease and renal recovery: consensus report of the Acute Disease Quality Initiative (ADQI) 16 Workgroup. Nat Rev Nephrol 2017;13(4):241–57.
3. Nixon AC, Bampouras TM, Pendleton N, et al. Frailty and chronic kidney disease: current evidence and continuing uncertainties. Clinical Kidney Journal 2018; 11(2):236–45.
4. Chowdhury R, Peel NM, Krosch M, et al. Frailty and chronic kidney disease: A systematic review. Arch Gerontol Geriatr 2017;68:135–42.
5. Ene-Iordache B, Perico N, Bikbov B, et al. Chronic kidney disease and cardiovascular risk in six regions of the world (ISN-KDDC): a cross-sectional study. Lancet Global Health 2016;4(5):e307–19.
6. Go AS, Chertow GM, Fan D, et al. Chronic Kidney Disease and the Risks of Death, Cardiovascular Events, and Hospitalization. N Engl J Med 2004; 351(13):1296–305.
7. Cockwell P, Fisher LA. The global burden of chronic kidney disease. Lancet 2020; 395(10225):662–4.

8. Global Burden of Disease Collaborative Network. Global Burden of. Disease Study 2019 (GBD 2019) Burden by Risk 1990-2019. Seattle, United States of America: Institute for Health Metrics and Evaluation (IHME; 2020. https://doi.org/10.6069/630D-5V32.

9. Johansen KL, Chertow GM, Foley RN, et al. US Renal Data System 2020 Annual Data Report: Epidemiology of Kidney Disease in the United States. Am J Kidney Dis 2021;77(4):A7–8.

10. Centers for Disease Control and Prevention. Chronic kidney disease in the United States, 2021. Atlanta, GA: US Department of Health and Human Services, Centers for Disease Control and Prevention; 2021.

11. Chu CD, McCulloch CE, Banerjee T, et al. CKD awareness among US adults by future risk of kidney failure. Am J Kidney Dis 2020;76(2):174–83.

12. Levin A, Stevens PE. Summary of KDIGO 2012 CKD Guideline: behind the scenes, need for guidance, and a framework for moving forward. Kidney Int 2014;85(1):49–61.

13. Smart NA, Titus TT. Outcomes of early versus late nephrology referral in chronic kidney disease: a systematic review. Am J Med 2011;124(11):1073–80.e2.

14. Kidney Disease Improving Global Outcomes (KDIGO). Chapter 5: Referral to specialists and models of care, Kidney Int Suppl 2013;3(1):112–9.

15. Cai Q, Mukku V, Ahmad M. Coronary artery disease in patients with chronic kidney disease: a clinical update. Cancer Chemother Rep 2014;9(4):331–9.

16. Perkovic V, de Zeeuw D, Mahaffey KW, et al. Canagliflozin and renal outcomes in type 2 diabetes: results from the CANVAS Program randomised clinical trials. Lancet Diabetes Endocrinol 2018;6(9):691–704.

17. Heerspink HJL, Stefansson BV, Correa-Rotter R, et al. Dapagliflozin in patients with chronic kidney disease. N Engl J Med 2020;383(15):1436–46.

18. Packer M, Anker SD, Butler J, et al. Cardiovascular and renal outcomes with empagliflozin in heart failure. N Engl J Med 2020;383(15):1413–24.

19. Pitt B, Filippatos G, Agarwal R, et al. Cardiovascular events with finerenone in kidney disease and type 2 diabetes. N Engl J Med 2021;385(24):2252–63.

20. Astor BC, Matsushita K, Gansevoort RT, et al. Lower estimated glomerular filtration rate and higher albuminuria are associated with mortality and end-stage renal disease. A collaborative meta-analysis of kidney disease population cohorts. Kidney Int 2011;79(12):1331–40.

21. Chronic Kidney Disease Prognosis Consortium, Matsushita K, van der Velde M, et al. Association of estimated glomerular filtration rate and albuminuria with all-cause and cardiovascular mortality in general population cohorts: a collaborative meta-analysis. Lancet 2010;375(9731):2073–81.

22. Bakris GL, Agarwal R, Anker SD, et al. Effect of finerenone on chronic kidney disease outcomes in type 2 diabetes. N Engl J Med 2020;383(23):2219–29.

23. The EMPA-KIDNEY Collaborative Group. Empagliflozin in patients with chronic kidney disease. N Engl J Med 2022. NEJMoa2204233.

24. Frampton JE. Finerenone: first approval. Drugs 2021;81(15):1787–94.

25. United States Renal Data System. USRDS annual data report: epidemiology of kidney disease in the United States. Bethesda, MD: National Institutes of Health, National Institute of Diabetes and Digestive and Kidney Diseases; 2022.

26. Stevens PE. Evaluation and management of chronic kidney disease: synopsis of the kidney disease: improving global outcomes 2012 clinical practice guideline. Ann Intern Med 2013;158(11):825.

27. Turin TC, Coresh J, Tonelli M, et al. One-year change in kidney function is associated with an increased mortality risk. Am J Nephrol 2012;36(1):41–9.

28. Turin TC, Coresh J, Tonelli M, et al. Short-term change in kidney function and risk of end-stage renal disease. Nephrol Dial Transplant 2012;27(10):3835–43.

29. Turin TC, Coresh J, Tonelli M, et al. Change in the estimated glomerular filtration rate over time and risk of all-cause mortality. Kidney Int 2013;83(4):684–91.

30. Kidney Disease. Improving Global Outcomes (KDIGO), Chapter 2: Definition, identification, and prediction of CKD progression. Kidney Int Suppl 2013;3(1): 63–72.

31. Lim DKE, Boyd JH, Thomas E, et al. Prediction models used in the progression of chronic kidney disease: A scoping review. In: Delanaye P, editor. PLoS One 2022; 17(7):e0271619.

32. Tangri N. A predictive model for progression of chronic kidney disease to kidney failure. JAMA 2011;305(15):1553.

33. Major RW, Shepherd D, Medcalf JF, et al. The kidney failure risk equation for prediction of end stage renal disease in uk primary care: an external validation and clinical impact projection cohort study. In: Rahimi K, editor. PLoS Med 2019; 16(11):e1002955.

34. Bundy JD, Mills KT, Anderson AH, et al. Prediction of end-stage kidney disease using estimated glomerular filtration rate with and without race: a prospective cohort study. Ann Intern Med 2022;175(3):305–13.

35. Kwek J, Pang H, Li H, et al. Validation of the kidney failure risk equation in predicting the risk of progression to kidney failure in a multi-ethnic Singapore chronic kidney disease cohort. smedj 2022;63(6):313–8.

36. Tangri N, Grams ME, Levey AS, et al. Multinational assessment of accuracy of equations for predicting risk of kidney failure: a meta-analysis. JAMA 2016; 315(2):164.

37. Norton JM, Moxey-Mims MM, Eggers PW, et al. Social determinants of racial disparities in CKD. JASN (J Am Soc Nephrol) 2016;27(9):2576–95.

38. Lorenz EC, Kennedy CC, Rule AD, et al. Frailty in CKD and Transplantation. Kidney International Reports 2021;6(9):2270–80.

39. Leung N, Bridoux F, Batuman V, et al. The evaluation of monoclonal gammopathy of renal significance: a consensus report of the International Kidney and Monoclonal Gammopathy Research Group. Nat Rev Nephrol 2019;15(1):45–59.

40. Korkmaz M, Aras B, Guneyli S, et al. Clinical significance of renal cortical thickness in patients with chronic kidney disease. Ultrasonography 2018;37(1):50–4.

41. Gupta P, Chatterjee S, Debnath J, et al. Ultrasonographic predictors in chronic kidney disease: A hospital based case control study. J Clin Ultrasound 2021; 49(7):715–9.

42. Argaiz ER, Koratala A, Reisinger N. Comprehensive assessment of fluid status by point-of-care ultrasonography. Kidney360 2021;2(8):1326–38.

43. Oliva-Damaso N, Oliva-Damaso E, Rodriguez-Perez JC, et al. Improved nephrology referral of chronic kidney disease patients: potential role of smartphone apps. Clinical Kidney Journal 2019;12(6):767–70.

44. Kottgen A, Cornec-Le Gall E, Halbritter J, et al. Genetics in chronic kidney disease: conclusions from a Kidney Disease: Improving Global Outcomes (KDIGO) Controversies Conference. Kidney Int 2022;101(6):1126–41.

45. Eckardt KU, Coresh J, Devuyst O, et al. Evolving importance of kidney disease: from subspecialty to global health burden. Lancet 2013;382(9887):158–69.

46. Rehberg PB. Studies on kidney function. Biochem J 1926;20(3):447–60.

47. Shannon JA, Smith HW. The excretion of inulin, xylose and urea by normal and phlorizinized man 1. J Clin Invest 1935;14(4):393–401.

48. Chasis H, Redish J, Goldring W, et al. The use of sodium p-aminohippurate for the functional evaluation of the human kidney 1. J Clin Invest 1945;24(4):583–8.
49. Smith H. The kidney: structure and function in health and disease. New York: Oxford University Press; 1951.
50. Stevens LA, Coresh J, Greene T, et al. Assessing kidney function — measured and estimated glomerular filtration rate. N Engl J Med 2006;354(23):2473–83.
51. Cockcroft DW, Gault H. Prediction of creatinine clearance from serum creatinine. Nephron 1976;16(1):31–41.
52. Myers GL. Recommendations for improving serum creatinine measurement: a report from the laboratory working group of the national kidney disease education program. Clin Chem 2006;52(1):5–18.
53. Delanaye P, White CA, Ebert N, et al. Assessing kidney function. In: Chronic renal disease. Elsevier; 2020. p. 37–54.
54. FDA. Guidance for Industry pharmacokinetics in patients with impaired renal function – study Design, data analysis, and impact on dosing. Published online September 2020. Available at: https://www.fda.gov/media/78573/download.
55. Levey AS. A more accurate method to estimate glomerular filtration rate from serum creatinine: a new prediction equation. Ann Intern Med 1999;130(6):461.
56. Levey AS, Stevens LA, Schmid CH, et al. A new equation to estimate glomerular filtration rate. Ann Intern Med 2009;150(9):604–12. Available at: https://www.ncbi.nlm.nih.gov/pmc/articles/PMC2763564/. Accessed July 22, 2020.
57. Inker LA, Schmid CH, Tighiouart H, et al. Estimating glomerular filtration rate from serum creatinine and cystatin C. N Engl J Med 2012. https://doi.org/10.1056/NEJMoa1114248.
58. Randers E, Erlandsen EJ. Serum cystatin c as an endogenous marker of the renal function – a Review. Clin Chem Lab Med 1999;37(4). https://doi.org/10.1515/CCLM.1999.064.
59. Delgado C, Baweja M, Crews DC, et al. A unifying approach for GFR estimation: recommendations of the NKF-ASN task force on reassessing the inclusion of race in diagnosing kidney disease. Am J Kidney Dis 2021. https://doi.org/10.1053/j.ajkd.2021.08.003. S0272638621008283.
60. Inker LA, Eneanya ND, Coresh J, et al. New creatinine- and cystatin c–based equations to estimate GFR without race. N Engl J Med 2021;385(19):1737–49.
61. Rule AD, Gussak HM, Pond GR, et al. Measured and estimated GFR in healthy potential kidney donors. Am J Kidney Dis 2004;43(1):112–9.
62. Hallan SI, Ritz E, Lydersen S, et al. Combining GFR and Albuminuria to Classify CKD Improves Prediction of ESRD. JASN (J Am Soc Nephrol) 2009;20(5):1069–77.
63. Zoja C, Abbate M, Remuzzi G. Progression of renal injury toward interstitial inflammation and glomerular sclerosis is dependent on abnormal protein filtration. Nephrol Dial Transplant 2015;30(5):706–12.
64. Lambers Heerspink HJ, Kropelin TF, Hoekman J, et al. Drug-Induced Reduction in Albuminuria Is Associated with Subsequent Renoprotection: A Meta-Analysis. JASN (J Am Soc Nephrol) 2015;26(8):2055–64.
65. Douville P, Martel AR, Talbot J, et al. Impact of age on glomerular filtration estimates. Nephrol Dial Transplant 2008;24(1):97–103.
66. Healthy people 2030, U.S. Department of Health and Human Services, Office of Disease Prevention and Health Promotion. Available at: https://health.gov/healthypeople/objectives-and-data/social-determinants-health.   Accessed December 10, 2022.

67. Lunyera J, Stanifer JW, Davenport CA, et al. Life Course Socioeconomic Status, Allostatic Load, and Kidney Health in Black Americans. CJASN 2020;15(3): 341–8.

68. Crews DC, Pfaff T, Powe NR. Socioeconomic Factors and Racial Disparities in Kidney Disease Outcomes. Semin Nephrol 2013;33(5):468–75.

69. Banerjee T, Crews DC, Wesson DE, et al. Food Insecurity, CKD, and Subsequent ESRD in US Adults. Am J Kidney Dis 2017;70(1):38–47.

70. Maziarz M, Chertow GM, Himmelfarb J, et al. Homelessness and risk of end-stage renal disease. J Health Care Poor Underserved 2014;25(3):1231–44.

71. Perez-Gomez MV, Martin-Cleary C, Fernandez-Fernandez B, et al. Meso-American nephropathy: what we have learned about the potential genetic influence on chronic kidney disease development. Clinical Kidney Journal 2018;11(4): 491–5.

72. Correa-Rotter R, Garcia-Trabanino R. Mesoamerican Nephropathy. Semin Nephrol 2019;39(3):263–71.

73. Genovese G, Friedman DJ, Ross MD, et al. Association of Trypanolytic ApoL1 Variants with Kidney Disease in African Americans. Science 2010;329(5993): 841–5.

74. Limou S, Nelson GW, Kopp JB, et al. APOL1 Kidney Risk Alleles: Population Genetics and Disease Associations. Adv Chron Kidney Dis 2014;21(5):426–33.

75. Kruzel-Davila E, Wasser WG, Aviram S, et al. APOL1 nephropathy: from gene to mechanisms of kidney injury. Nephrol Dial Transplant 2016;31(3):349–58.

76. Nasr SH, Kopp JB. COVID-19–Associated Collapsing Glomerulopathy: An Emerging Entity. Kidney International Reports 2020;5(6):759–61.

77. Kasembeli AN, Duarte R, Ramsay M, et al. APOL1 Risk Variants Are Strongly Associated with HIV-Associated Nephropathy in Black South Africans. J Am Soc Nephrol 2015;26(11):2882.

78. Lipkowitz MS, Freedman BI, Langefeld CD, et al. Apolipoprotein L1 gene variants associate with hypertension-attributed nephropathy and the rate of kidney function decline in African Americans. Kidney Int 2013;83(1):114–20.

79. Stevens LA, Levey AS. Measured GFR as a Confirmatory Test for Estimated GFR. J Am Soc Nephrol 2009;20(11):2305–13.

Urinalysis
Interpretation and Clinical Correlations

Kanza Haq, MD, Dipal M. Patel, MD, PhD*

KEYWORDS

- Urinalysis • Proteinuria • Hematuria • Glucosuria • Ketonuria • Crystalluria
- Nephrolithiasis

KEY POINTS

- Urinalyses are commonly ordered and widely available, and are a powerful tool to help understand potential pathologies related to the kidney and urinary systems.
- Urine samples have several physical and chemical properties that can be relevant to clinical scenarios.
- Urine microscopy can reveal evidence of conditions including glomerular disease, intrinsic kidney injury, nephrolithiasis, or drug-induced crystalluria.
- Concomitant urinalysis with bloodwork is a key initial step in diagnosing glomerular diseases.

INTRODUCTION

Urinalysis is an invaluable, noninvasive diagnostic test that is commonly used in clinical practice in both inpatient and ambulatory settings. Correct interpretation of urine studies in conjunction with a patient's history, physical examination, and laboratory data can provide clinicians with crucial information about a wide variety of primary kidney and systemic disorders, even in asymptomatic patients.[1,2] This review serves to summarize the interpretation of various patterns of urinalysis findings. We aim to aid primary care and internal medicine physicians in using urinalysis to (1) evaluate suspected acute and chronic kidney diseases, (2) monitor the course of established diseases, and (3) refine the differential diagnosis and optimize further workup in settings of unknown disease pathology.

DEFINITIONS

- Spot urine collection: a small sample of urine from a single voiding event
- Timed urine collection: a sample of urine collected from multiple voiding events over a specified time period (typically 24 hours)

Division of Nephrology, Department of Internal Medicine, Johns Hopkins University, 1830 East Monument Street, Suite 416, Baltimore, MD 21287, USA
* Corresponding author.
E-mail address: dpatel85@jhmi.edu

Med Clin N Am 107 (2023) 659–679
https://doi.org/10.1016/j.mcna.2023.03.002
medical.theclinics.com

- Urine microscopy: examination of urine elements under a microscope to detect the presence of various cells, casts, and crystals
- Proteinuria: the presence of elevated levels of proteins in the urine, which can include albumin as well as other serum proteins such as globulins
- Albuminuria: the presence of elevated levels of albumin in the urine
- Acute kidney injury (AKI): increase in serum creatinine by $\geq$0.3 mg/dL within 48 hours, increase in serum creatinine by >1.5× baseline, or urine volume <0.5 mL/kg/h over a 6-hour period[3]
- Chronic kidney disease (CKD): persistently impaired estimated glomerular filtration rate <60 mL/min/1.73 m^2 or persistently elevated urine albumin excretion $\geq$30 mg/g creatinine, or both, for more than 3 months[3]

When Should Urinalysis Be Pursued?

Urinalysis is a simple and inexpensive test that can be performed in many clinical situations. There is currently insufficient evidence to support universal urinalysis screening.[4–6] We recommend urinalysis for the following patients.

1. Any patient with an elevated serum creatinine level, in the evaluation of either AKI or CKD
2. Patients with diabetes, hypertension, or cardiovascular disease[7,8]
3. Patients with new or unexplained progressive edema
4. Patients being evaluated for certain systemic diseases with renal manifestations, such as lupus, vasculitis, or monoclonal gammopathies
5. Patients presenting with symptoms or clinical evidence of nephrolithiasis
6. Patients with concerns of discolored urine, frothy urine, or symptoms consistent with urinary tract infections (UTIs)

How Should a Urine Specimen Be Collected?

In most clinical situations, investigation of urine begins with a spot collection. Proper collection and handling of urine specimens is important to maximize the diagnostic yield and achieve reliable interpretation of findings. Midstream clean-catch collections are preferred to reduce cellular and microbial contamination from skin flora. Early morning samples are optimal, as urine accumulated overnight is more concentrated and contains relatively higher levels of cellular elements and proteins, which can be missed in dilute samples.[9] Early morning samples can also provide more reliable information about a patient's urine concentrating capacity.

During evaluation of specific conditions such as glomerular disease, monoclonal gammopathies, or nephrolithiasis, collection of 24-hour urine samples may be warranted. Patients should be instructed to discard their first morning void and subsequently collect all urine produced over the following 24 hours.[10]

In patients with an indwelling urinary catheter, fresh samples should be taken from the side port of the catheter, as this represents recently produced urine. Samples taken from collection bags can be affected by precipitation and contamination and are considered inaccurate. If a patient is undergoing evaluation for a possible UTI, indwelling catheters should first be replaced, with a urine sample and culture sent from the fresh catheter.[11]

Samples from patients with nephrostomy tubes should ideally be obtained at the time of tube placement. For patients who already have a nephrostomy tube in place, the drainage bag should be changed, and a subsequently produced urine sample should drain by gravity into a sterile collection container. Urostomy samples are recommended to be collected by transiently catheterizing the stoma and collecting the first subsequent void. Specimens should not be collected from the urostomy pouch or drainage bag, as both will contain significant contamination.[12,13]

How Should Specimens Be Handled?

Once a spot sample is collected, urinalysis should be performed within 2 to 4 hours, as delays between collection and examination can influence results due to instability of some urinary components and overgrowth of clinically significant or contaminating flora.[14,15] Samples processed outside of this timeframe may be affected by alterations in cellular morphology and the development of cellular casts or crystals that have developed *ex vivo*. If a specimen cannot be examined promptly, such as a 24-hour timed urine collection, it should be refrigerated at a temperature of 2°C to 8°C for up to 24 to 48 hours.[16,17] Storage at cold temperatures can still result in some inaccuracies due to decomposition and/or precipitation of phosphates and urates.

What Methods Can Be Used to Analyze a Urine Sample?

A urinalysis, also referred to as a urine dipstick test, uses a plastic strip with attached chemical reagent pads for pH, protein, glucose, ketone, bilirubin, urobilinogen, blood, nitrite, and leukocyte esterase. The dipstick can be analyzed manually based on visual color changes to the various reagent pads, or placed into an automated reader, which is the standard for a urinalysis examination in a clinical laboratory. This testing method comes with some limitations stemming from common false-positive and false-negative results.[18] A urine microscopy test to visualize cells, casts, and crystals is typically done as a secondary test when abnormalities are found on the initial urinalysis.

What Are the Commonly Reported Properties of Urine?

A urinalysis consists of three components (**Table 1**): physical properties, chemical properties, and elements identified by microscopic examination.[18–20] Each of these components can provide unique insight into the pathology of a patient's kidney or urologic conditions.

- Color: Normal urine is clear with a light/pale yellow tinge due to the presence of urochrome generated from heme breakdown. Urine color can be affected by a

Table 1 Properties of urinalysis	
Physical examination	Color Odor Turbidity Specific gravity
Chemical examination	pH Protein Glucose Urobilinogen, bilirubin Ketone bodies Leukocyte esterase Nitrites
Microscopic examination	Cells Casts Crystals Microorganisms

Characteristics obtained from physical, chemical, and microscopic examinations are listed.

variety of normal or pathological conditions, metabolic products, medications, foods, drugs, and infections[18–25] (**Table 2**).

- Odor: Urine odor can be altered by certain clinical conditions, foods, bacteria, and drugs[18–20] (**Table 3**).
- Turbidity: While urine is normally clear or transparent, turbidity can be reported in settings of crystal precipitation after refrigeration, or with the presence of erythrocytes, blood clots, leukocytes, bacteria, squamous epithelial cells, vaginal secretions, semen, or chyluria.[18–20]
- Volume: In adults, urine volume ranges from 600 mL to 2000 mL over 24 hours, on average. Patients with <100 mL of urine per day are deemed anuric, whereas oliguric patients produce <500 mL/day. Polyuria is suspected when urine output exceeds 3000 mL over 24 hours in adults and can be seen in conditions such as diabetes mellitus, diabetes insipidus, psychogenic polydipsia, diuretic use, or excess alcohol or caffeine consumption.[26,27] In the nonacute setting, 24-hour urine volumes can be useful to objectively assess for polyuria or to determine if hydration status might be a contributing risk factor for nephrolithiasis.
- Specific gravity (s.g.): The urine s.g. measures the concentration of solutes (number and size of particles) in urine. The range is dependent on the amount of fluid ingested and solute excreted. If urine does not contain glucose, proteins, or large molecules such as contrast media, the urine osmolality can be inferred from urine s.g. (urine s.g. of 1.001–1.035 corresponds to urine osmolality of 50–1200 mOsm/kg). Indirectly, urine s.g. can provide information on urinary concentrating and diluting capabilities and can be helpful in evaluation of volume disorders, as well as disorders of water balance such as hyponatremia or hypernatremia.[28]
  - High urine s.g. is seen in cases of volume depletion, syndrome of inappropriate antidiuretic hormone, and glucosuria. It can also be induced with administration of hyperosmotic solutions including iodinated contrast, IV albumin, and dextran.
  - A urine s.g. of 1.010 is isotonic to plasma (isosthenuria).
  - Urine s.g. <1.010 indicates urinary dilution and can be seen in conditions including excessive fluid intake, psychogenic polydipsia, and diabetes insipidus. A urine s.g. ≤1.003 indicates maximally dilute urine.
- Urine pH: Urine pH reflects the degree of acidification of urine. Physiologic urine pH ranges from 4.5 to 8 depending on systemic acid-base balance. On a typical Western diet, urine is slightly acidic (pH 5.5–6.5) because of metabolic activity, which predominantly favors acid formation. Determination of urine pH is useful in the diagnosis and management of nephrolithiasis, metabolic acidosis, and UTIs (**Table 4**) and provides insight into tubular function. Low urine pH can be seen in patients with high-protein diets, systemic acidosis, type IV renal tubular acidosis (RTA), and heavy intake of certain fruits and medications (e.g., cranberries ormethionine). High urine pH can be seen in patients following a strict vegetarian diet, patients with systemic alkalosis, UTIs caused by urease-producing organisms, or type I RTA.[19] Changes in urine pH may also be helpful in management of drug toxicities requiring urinary alkalinization, such as methotrexate, salicylate, phenobarbital, and chlorpropamide toxicity.[29]
- Hematuria: Hematuria can be gross (visible to the naked eye) or microscopic (detectable only on urinalysis). Microscopic hematuria refers to the presence of 3 or more erythrocytes per high-powered field.
  - Dipsticks are very sensitive to urinary hemoglobin, which can be free or seen within red blood cells (RBCs). Dipsticks detect the peroxidase activity of erythrocytes, which is also catalyzed by myoglobin and hemoglobin; therefore, a positive test result may indicate hematuria, myoglobinuria, or hemoglobinuria.

Table 2
Urine color

Color	Conditions	Drugs/Substances	Foods
Dark yellow	Concentrated urine in dehydration or exercise	Vitamin preparations, rifampin	Carrots
Pink/red	Hematuria, hemoglobin, myoglobin, porphyrin, massive uric acid crystalluria	Phenothiazines	Beets, blackberries, rhubarb
Orange	Bilirubin, bile pigments	Phenazopyridine, vitamin C, rifampin, phenothiazines, warfarin	Carrots
Green/blue	Pseudomonas UTI	Cimetidine, propofol, amitriptyline, biliverdin, promethazine (Phenergan), triamterene, cimetidine, methylene blue, and indigo dyes	Asparagus
Purple	Infection with Escherichia coli or Pseudomonas, bacteriuria from indwelling catheter	Hydroxocobalamin	
Black/brown/tea colored	Bile pigments, myoglobinuria, methemoglobin, melanuria, porphyria, homogentisic acid (alkaptonuria)	Chloroquine, levodopa, methyldopa, nitrofurantoin	Rhubarb
Cloudy/white	Pyuria, chyle, calcium phosphate crystals, struvite crystals	Propofol	

Conditions, drugs, substances, and foods associated with different urine colors are shown.[18-25]

Table 3
Urine odor may be affected by a variety of substances or conditions, as shown[18–20]

Odor	Substances or Conditions
Strong smell	Concentrated urine, dehydration, old specimen
Fruity or sweet odor	Acetone in diabetic ketoacidosis
Ammoniac	Alkaline fermentation after prolonged bladder retention, UTI by urease-producing organisms
Pungent	UTI, asparagus consumption
Fecal	Gastrointestinal bladder fistula
Burnt sugar/maple syrup	Maple syrup urine disease
Mousy/musty odor	Phenylketonuria
Sulfur	Asparagus, sulfa medications

Microscopic examination of the urine sediment is the gold standard for detection of hematuria and may also identify RBC casts or dysmorphic RBCs.

- ○ Hematuria is divided into glomerular, nonglomerular, and urologic etiologies.
  - ■ Glomerular hematuria can be associated with dysmorphic RBCs, erythrocyte casts, and proteinuria, and can be seen in conditions such as IgA nephropathy, type IV collagen diseases, thin basement membrane disease, or various nephritic diseases. Patients with glomerular hematuria should be referred to nephrology for further evaluation.
  - ■ Nonglomerular hematuria can be associated with proteinuria, without dysmorphic RBCs or erythrocyte casts. Nonglomerular hematuria can be seen in patients with tubulointerstitial disease, polycystic kidney disease, sickle cell disease, or papillary necrosis. A subclass of nonglomerular hematuria is urologic hematuria, which can be associated with passage of clots. Patients with urologic hematuria should be referred for further evaluation of etiologies such as nephrolithiasis, malignancies, benign prostatic hyperplasia, or lower UTIs.[30]

- Proteinuria: Proteinuria is a very common finding and can arise from several different physiologic and pathologic causes. The presence and degree of proteinuria, especially albuminuria, is important for CKD staging and the prognostication of progression.[31,32] Proteins <20,000 Da pass easily across the glomerular capillary wall; however, the negatively charged large protein albumin (69,000 Da) is repelled by the glomerular capillary wall and normally present in only small

Table 4
Analysis of urine pH

Nephrolithiasis	• Urine pH < 5.5: uric acid stones • Urine pH > 6.5: calcium phosphate stones
Metabolic acidosis	• Urine pH < 5.5: Type IV RTA (hyperkalemic distal RTA) • Urine pH > 5.5: Type I RTA (hypokalemic distal RTA) • Type II (proximal) RTA initially results in alkaline urine due to an inability to reabsorb bicarbonate, but urine later becomes acidic as the filtered load of bicarbonate decreases.
UTIs	• Urine pH > 7.0: UTI secondary to urease-producing organisms

Urine pH can guide evaluation of conditions including nephrolithiasis, metabolic acidosis, and UTIs.

Abbreviation: RTA, renal tubular acidosis.

amounts in glomerular filtrate.[32] Most smaller-molecular-weight filtered proteins are largely reabsorbed and metabolized primarily in proximal convoluted tubules, with only small amounts excreted. Tamm-Horsfall glycoprotein is secreted by tubular cells and comprises 40% to 50% of total urinary proteins, with the rest being primarily made of albumin and globulins.

○ Some patients may experience transient proteinuria, which can occur due to temporary changes in glomerular hemodynamics and usually resolves as the precipitating factor is addressed. Some causes of benign transient proteinuria are dehydration, exposure to extreme heat or cold, emotional stress, fever, inflammatory processes, UTIs, acute illnesses, vaginal mucus, heavy exercise, or orthostatic changes (postural proteinuria).

○ On the other hand, persistent proteinuria or albuminuria suggests the presence of kidney disease and can be divided into three categories[32,33]:

▪ Glomerular proteinuria is the most common cause of proteinuria and occurs as a result of altered permeability of a damaged glomerular basement membrane, causing urinary loss of large-molecular-weight proteins such as albumin and immunoglobulins. In many cases, glomerular proteinuria is further quantified by assessing albuminuria, which is classified into three stages[34]: A1 (less than 30 mg/g creatinine; normal to mildly increased), A2 (30 mg/g to 300 mg/g creatinine; moderately increased, "microalbuminuria"), and A3 (greater than 300 mg/g creatinine; severely increased, "macroalbuminuria").

▪ Tubular proteinuria results from an inability of malfunctioning tubular cells to metabolize or reabsorb normally filtered low-molecular-weight proteins (e.g., retinol-binding protein, α-2-microglobulin, β-2-microglobulin). Tubular proteinuria is typically <2 g/d.

▪ Overflow proteinuria occurs when low-molecular-weight proteins (e.g., myoglobin, immunoglobulin light chains) are overproduced, thereby overwhelming the ability of the tubules to reabsorb all filtered proteins.

○ Proteinuria can be further classified as subnephrotic range (150–3000 mg per day) or nephrotic range (>3500 mg per day). This classification helps narrow potential disease etiologies (**Table 5**).

Table 5
Potential disease etiologies by degree of proteinuria

Nephrotic range proteinuria (>3500 mg/d)	• Diabetic nephropathy • Focal segmental glomerulosclerosis • Minimal change disease • Membranous nephropathy • Amyloidosis • Dysproteinemia (e.g., multiple myeloma)
Subnephrotic proteinuria (150–3000 mg/d)	• IgA nephropathy • Type IV collagen diseases (e.g., thin basement membrane disease) • Lupus nephritis • Infection-related GN • Membranoproliferative GN • Anti-GBM disease • ANCA vasculitis • Acute interstitial nephritis

Several disease etiologies can present with variable proteinuria levels.
Abbreviations: GBM, glomerular basement membrane; GN, glomerulonephritis; ANCA, antineutrophilic cytoplasmic antibody.

- Nephrotic range proteinuria is seen in primary glomerular diseases (e.g., minimal change disease or membranous nephropathy), but can also be seen in cases of overflow proteinuria (e.g., multiple myeloma). When nephrotic range proteinuria is associated with hypoalbuminemia and edema, it is called nephrotic syndrome. Patients with nephrotic syndrome should be referred for prompt nephrology evaluation.
- Subnephrotic range proteinuria can be seen in settings of glomerular (e.g., glomerulonephritis) or nonglomerular parenchymal renal disease (e.g., tubulointerstitial or vascular processes).
- Many disease pathologies can present with variable degrees of proteinuria. Regardless, patients with unexplained proteinuria, or progressive proteinuria with hematuria, should be evaluated by a nephrologist.

Proteinuria may be quantified by several different approaches:

o Urine dipstick: A standard urine dipstick test is the most common first-line screening tool for proteinuria. The reagent on most dipstick tests is sensitive to albumin, with 1+ corresponding to 30 mg/dL, 2+ to 100 mg/dL, 3+ to 300 mg/dL, and 4+ to 1,000 mg/dL albuminuria. Urine dipstick testing is usually highly specific for detecting proteinuria but has lower sensitivity.[35] False results can occur in situations of varied urine concentration. Positive results may be seen in dehydrated patients with highly concentrated urine, patients who have received iodinated radiocontrast agents, patients who have recently exercised, or patients with gross hematuria, alkaline urine, or a UTI. Very dilute urine can also result in false-negative results.

- Another significant limitation of urine dipsticks is low sensitivity to nonalbumin proteins, such as light chain immunoglobulins and Bence-Jones proteins.[36] This problem can be addressed by performing the sulfosalicylic acid (SSA) test, which is a semiquantitative method available to screen patients for proteinuria. The SSA test reagent detects all proteins in urine including immunoglobulins.[36] When the SSA test is positive with a negative dipstick, it usually indicates the presence of nonalbumin proteins in the urine. As neither dipstick nor the SSA method is quantitative, more formal urinalysis testing should be pursued if one of the described tests is positive.

o 24-hour urine protein excretion: The gold standard to quantify proteinuria is a 24-hour urine collection, as it eliminates variations in proteinuria associated with the circadian rhythm and can also be standardized to a 24-hour urine creatinine. There are certain limitations to this approach, mostly surrounding methods and difficulty of collection. It can be impractical and cumbersome in outpatient settings or in care of older patients, and is susceptible to overcollection (urine collected for >24 hours) or undercollection (urine collected for <24 hours), which can influence results.

o Spot urine albumin-to-creatinine ratio (UACR) and urine protein-to-creatinine ratio (UPCR): An alternative to 24-hour urine protein excretion is quantification of the UPCR or UACR, both of which use a spot urine sample. UACR and UPCR are more accurate than urine dipsticks and correlate well with 24-hour collections in adults.[37] This approach is also easier for patients and standardizes the protein measurement to the quantity of creatinine in the urine, which helps avoid errors introduced by dilute or concentrated urine samples. Major limitations to UPCR and UACR are overestimation or underestimation of proteinuria in individuals with small or large muscle mass, respectively, as it is influenced by urine creatinine. Correlations of

Table 6
Cellular elements identified on urine microscopy[41-46]

Cell Type	Characteristics	Causes	Representative Image
Epithelial cells	*Renal tubular epithelial (RTE) cells* are larger than PMNs and have a round, large, centrally located nucleus and fine-grained cytoplasm.	Tubular damage, interstitial nephritis	
	Squamous epithelial cells are derived from the distal urethra or external genitalia. They are large and irregular with a small nucleus and fine granular cytoplasm.	Contamination during sample collection	

(continued on next page)

Table 6
(continued)

Cell Type	Characteristics	Causes	Representative Image
	Transitional epithelial cells originate from the renal pelvis, ureter, bladder, or proximal urethra. They are smaller and rounder than squamous cells and have larger nuclei.	Contamination during sample collection, transitional cell cancers	
White blood cells[41]	*Neutrophils* are intermediate in size compared with RBCs and renal tubular epithelial cells. They have an agranular cytoplasm and multilobed nuclei.	Urinary tract inflammation or infection, bacteriuria, interstitial nephritis, genitourinary tuberculosis, nephrolithiasis	
	Urine eosinophils can be detected with Wright or Hansel stain to the urine sediment.	Urine eosinophils are found in a variety of kidney diseases. They are not accurate to establish or exclude a diagnosis of acute interstitial nephritis.[42–44]	

Erythrocytes[45,46]	*Isomorphic RBCs* are small, enucleated cells shaped as biconcave discs.	Nonglomerular hematuria
	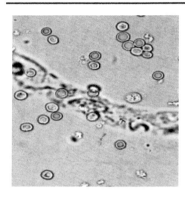	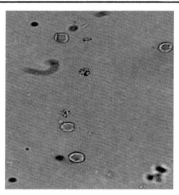
	Dysmorphic RBCs have variable shapes because of their passage through the glomerulus. Acanthocytes are RBCs with membrane protrusions.	Glomerular hematuria (52% sensitivity and 98% specificity for diagnosis of glomerulonephritis)

Arthur Greenberg, 4 - Urinalysis and Urine Microscopy, Editor(s): Scott J. Gilbert, Daniel E. Weiner, National Kidney Foundation Primer on Kidney Diseases (Sixth Edition), W.B. Saunders, 2014, Pages 33-41, https://doi.org/10.1016/B978-1-4557-4617-0.00004-2.

Table 7
Cellular and acellular casts identified on urine microscopy

Casts	Composition	Conditions	Representative Image
Hyaline	Solidified Tamm-Horsfall mucoprotein	Nonspecific; can be seen in concentrated urine from healthy individuals, or in settings of fever, physical exertion, or chronic renal disease	
Erythrocyte	Red blood cells in a tubular cast matrix	Glomerulonephritis, interstitial nephritis; also seen as a normal finding (along with hematuria) in healthy individuals after exercise	
Leukocyte	White blood cells in a tubular cast matrix	Pyelonephritis, interstitial nephritis	

| Epithelial | Renal tubular cells in a tubular cast matrix | Acute tubular necrosis, interstitial nephritis; can also be seen in concentrated urine | 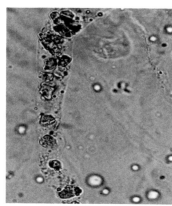 |
| Granular | Fine or coarse casts composed of cellular breakdown products, within a cast matrix | Acute tubular necrosis; also seen in other etiologies such as glomerulonephritis or tubulointerstitial disease | 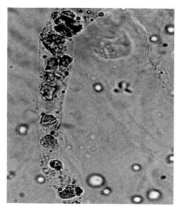 |

(continued on next page)

Table 7
(continued)

Casts	Composition	Conditions	Representative Image
Waxy	Hyaline material and proteinaceous material	Nonspecific; seen in advanced CKD and AKI	
Fatty	Lipid-laden renal tubular epithelial cells	Nephrotic syndrome	

Arthur Greenberg. 4 - Urinalysis and Urine Microscopy. Editor(s): Scott J. Gilbert, Daniel E. Weiner, National Kidney Foundation Primer on Kidney Diseases (Sixth Edition), W.B. Saunders, 2014, Pages 33–41, https://doi.org/10.1016/B978-1-4557-4617-0.00004-2.

Table 8
Crystals identified on urine microscopy

Type of Crystal	Shape	Urine pH	Associations	Figure
Cystine	Hexagonal shapes similar to benzene rings	Acidic	Cystinuria	
Calcium oxalate	Envelope or dumbbell	Acidic	High dietary oxalate, nephrolithiasis, ethylene glycol ingestion	
Uric acid	Diamond, barrel, rhomboid, or needle-shaped	Acidic, typically with urine pH < 5.5	Urate nephrolithiasis, acute urate nephropathy; less common in normal subjects	
Triple phosphate (magnesium ammonium phosphate)	Coffin lid	Alkaline	Nephrolithiasis, UTIs secondary to urease-producing organisms (*Proteus*, *Klebsiella*)	

Arthur Greenberg, 4 - Urinalysis and Urine Microscopy, Editor(s): Scott J. Gilbert, Daniel E. Weiner, National Kidney Foundation Primer on Kidney Diseases (Sixth Edition), W.B. Saunders, 2014, Pages 33–41, https://doi.org/10.1016/B978-1-4557-4617-0.00004-2.

spot samples with 24-hour protein excretion are less robust in patients with nephrotic-range proteinuria and in patients who are pregnant.[37]

- Glucosuria: Glucosuria occurs when the filtered load of glucose exceeds the re-absorbing capacity of the tubule, or if the kidney is unable to reabsorb filtered glucose despite normal plasma glucose concentrations.[20] Glucosuria is classically a feature of diabetes and can be seen in Cushing syndrome. Glucosuria in the absence of hyperglycemia suggests proximal tubular dysfunction, which can be seen in multiple myeloma, cast nephropathies, or heavy metal exposure, or due to exposure to certain drugs such as sodium/glucose cotransporter-2 inhibitors, valproic acid, aminoglycosides, cisplatin, and tenofovir.[19]

- Ketonuria: Ketones are products of body fat metabolism. Ketonuria is seen in diabetic acidosis, alcoholic acidosis, starvation, and pregnancy. As the urine dipstick reagent detects the reaction of nitroprusside with acetoacetate and acetone, it underestimates ketone excretion in diabetic ketoacidosis or starvation ketosis, which primarily generate β-hydroxybutyrate.[19]

- Leukocyte esterase: Leukocyte esterase is produced by lysed neutrophils and macrophages and is a surrogate marker for the presence of white blood cells. Proteinuria, glucosuria, ketonuria, and certain drugs such as cephalosporins, nitrofurantoin, tetracycline, or gentamicin can lead to a false-negative leukocyte esterase test. False-positive results are rare but can be seen in contaminated urine samples or in samples mixed with vaginal secretions.

- Nitrites: A positive urine nitrite test indicates the presence of bacteria that are capable of reducing urinary nitrates into nitrites via the nitrate reductase enzyme. Many gram-negative bacteria and some gram-positive organisms (E. coli, Klebsiella, Enterobacter, Citrobacter, Klebsiella, and Proteus species) have this capability. The presence of both leukocyte esterase and nitrites on urine dipstick is highly predictive of a UTI.[38] Urinary infections with species that express low levels of nitrate reductase (Pseudomonas, Staphylococcus, and Enterococcus species) may test negative for nitrites.

- Bilirubin and urobilinogen: Conjugated bilirubin is not normally present in urine in detectable amounts but can be positive in patients with hepatic or biliary

Table 9
Common urinalysis findings with respective likely etiologies

Urinalysis Findings	Likely Etiology
Bland or hyaline casts, few finely granular casts; ± protein	Prerenal azotemia
"Muddy brown" casts, RTE cells or casts; ± protein	Acute tubular injury
Dysmorphic RBCs, RBC casts, subnephrotic proteinuria	Nephritic syndrome
Fatty casts, cholesterol crystals, oval fat bodies, nephrotic-range proteinuria	Nephrotic syndrome
Urine glucose in the absence of hyperglycemia	SGLT2i use; proximal tubular dysfunction from multiple myeloma or cast nephropathies
Urine specific gravity >1.035	Radiographic contrast use; volume depletion
Urine pH > 6 in the setting of systemic non-anion-gap metabolic acidosis	RTA (likely type 1)

Abbreviations: RTE, renal tubular epithelial; SGLT2i, sodium/glucose cotransporter-2 inhibitor.

Table 10
Common clinical scenarios

Clinical Scenario	Urinalysis Findings	Likely Diagnosis	Next Steps
65-year-old male with a 5-year history of diabetes (A1c 7.5%–9.0%); Cr 1.1 mg/dL	UACR 220 mg/g; UPCR 0.4 g/g	Early diabetic nephropathy	Initiation of RASi, SGLT2i, GLP1-RA; monitoring of albuminuria every 6 mo; nephrology referral with worsening of proteinuria or Cr.
23-year-old male with hematuria and recent respiratory infection; Cr 1.1 mg/dL	3+ blood, 2+ protein; UPCR 1.2 mg/g	IgA nephropathy, postinfectious GN	Nephrology referral (possible kidney biopsy)
32-year-old female with mild anemia and hypercalcemia; Cr 1.3 mg/dL	Dipstick negative for protein, but with ++SSA; UPCR 4.3 g/g; UACR 0.5 mg/g	Dysproteinemia (myeloma, amyloidosis, cast nephropathy)	Nephrology referral (possible kidney biopsy); hematology referral (possible bone marrow biopsy)
75-year-old male with rapid-onset anasarca; Cr 0.9 mg/dL	UPCR 12.2 g/g; UACR 6000 mg/g	Minimal change disease, membranous nephropathy	Nephrology referral (kidney biopsy)
78-year-old male with 1-mo history of intermittent gross hematuria and blood clots, urinary frequency, nocturia; Cr 1.1	2+ blood on dipstick; no dysmorphic RBCs or RBC casts on urine sediment	Urological malignancy, benign prostatic hyperplasia	Urology referral (cystoscopy)
30-year-old male with 1 episode of transient macroscopic hematuria and flank pain; Cr 1.2	+ blood on dipstick; 10–15 isomorphic erythrocytes on urine sediment	Nephrolithiasis	Noncontrast computed tomography or ultrasound; 24-h urine collection for stone risk panel

Urinalysis findings can help formulate differential diagnoses.
Abbreviations: Cr, creatinine; GLP1-RA, glucagon-like peptide-1 receptor agonists; GN, glomerulonephritis; RASi, renin-angiotensin system inhibitor; SGLT2i, sodium/glucose cotransporter-2 inhibitor.

obstruction or congenital hyperbilirubinemia.[20] This test is usually negative in patients with jaundice due to hemolysis, as unconjugated bilirubin is fat soluble.

Urobilinogen is the end product of conjugated bilirubin metabolism and is present in urine in only small amounts. Elevated levels suggest an excess of conjugated or unconjugated bilirubin, which can be seen in cases of hemolysis and hepatocellular diseases like cirrhosis and hepatitis. Certain antibiotics (e.g., sulfonamides) may produce false-positive results, and exposure of urine samples to daylight or prolonged storage can cause false-negative results due to degradation of urobilinogen.[20]

What Additional Information Is Offered by Urine Microscopy?

Urine microscopic examination is an indispensable part of the evaluation of patients with hematuria, proteinuria, or nephrolithiasis. To perform urine microscopy, a fresh sample of 10–15 mL of urine is centrifuged for at least 5 minutes at >1500 rpm. The supernatant is then poured out, and the sediment is resuspended with gentle shaking of the tube. A single drop of urine sediment is placed on a glass slide and examined under a microscope. Although automated microscopic platforms have been developed to identify cells and particles in urine, the diagnostic yield may be substantially greater when it is performed by a clinician trained in urine microscopy.[39,40] Urine microscopy can primarily be used to evaluate cellular structures (**Table 6**), casts (**Table 7**), and crystals (**Table 8**). While routine use of urine microscopy is not anticipated in non-nephrology settings, a basic understanding of the impact of urine microscopy in clinical diagnosis and management of patients is important.

SUMMARY

Urinalysis is a powerful tool and can be integral to the clinical evaluation of patients with kidney diseases (**Tables 9** and **10**). Correct acquisition of the sample and interpretation of findings within the context of the clinical situation can not only provide valuable information to internists but also guide next steps in diagnostic and therapeutic interventions.

CLINICS CARE POINTS

- Urinalysis should be performed in patients with acute or chronic kidney injury, evidence of kidney stones, change in urine appearance, or urinary symptoms.
- Proper collection and handling of urine specimens is key to reliability of findings.
- Patients with hypertension, diabetes mellitus, or cardiovascular disease should be screened for proteinuria.
- The presence and degree of proteinuria (especially albuminuria) is important for chronic kidney disease (CKD) staging and prognostication and should be monitored at regular intervals for patients with proteinuric CKD.
- Glucosuria in the absence of hyperglycemia suggests proximal tubular dysfunction, which can be seen in multiple myeloma and cast nephropathies, or due to exposure to certain drugs such as sodium/glucose cotransporter-2 inhibitors.
- Unexplained persistent proteinuria or hematuria, and nephrotic range proteinuria, warrant further investigation including consideration of referral to nephrology.

DISCLOSURE

The authors have nothing to disclose.

REFERENCES

1. Fogazzi GB, Verdesca S, Garigali G. Urinalysis: core curriculum 2008. Am J Kidney Dis 2008;51(6):1052–67.
2. Cavanaugh C, Perazella MA. Urine Sediment Examination in the Diagnosis and Management of Kidney Disease: Core Curriculum 2019. Am J Kidney Dis 2019; 73(2):258–72.
3. Khwaja A. KDIGO clinical practice guidelines for acute kidney injury. Nephron Clin Pract 2012;120(4):c179–84.
4. Moyer VA, U.S. Preventive Services Task Force. Screening for chronic kidney disease: U.S. Preventive Services Task Force recommendation statement. Ann Intern Med 2012;157(8):567–70.
5. Fink HA, Ishani A, Taylor BC, et al. Screening for, monitoring, and treatment of chronic kidney disease stages 1 to 3: a systematic review for the U.S. Preventive Services Task Force and for an American College of Physicians Clinical Practice Guideline. Ann Intern Med 2012;156(8):570–81.
6. Samal L, Linder JA. The primary care perspective on routine urine dipstick screening to identify patients with albuminuria. Clin J Am Soc Nephrol 2013; 8(1):131–5.
7. Shlipak MG, Tummalapalli SL, Boulware LE, et al. The case for early identification and intervention of chronic kidney disease: conclusions from a Kidney Disease: Improving Global Outcomes (KDIGO) Controversies Conference. Kidney Int 2021;99(1):34–47.
8. American Diabetes Association Professional Practice Committee, Draznin B, Aroda VR, et al. 11. Chronic Kidney Disease and Risk Management: Standards of Medical Care in Diabetes-2022. Diabetes Care 2022;45(Suppl 1):S175–84.
9. European Confederation of Laboratory Medicine. European urinalysis guidelines. Scand J Clin Lab Invest Suppl 2000;231:1–86.
10. Corder CJ, Rathi BM, Sharif S, Leslie SW. 24-Hour Urine Collection. 2022. In: StatPearls [Internet]. Treasure Island (FL): StatPearls; 2023.
11. McGoldrick M. Urine specimen collection and transport. Home Healthc Now 2015;33(5):284–5.
12. Mahoney M, Baxter K, Burgess J, et al. Procedure for obtaining a urine sample from a urostomy, ileal conduit, and colon conduit: a best practice guideline for clinicians. J Wound, Ostomy Cont Nurs 2013;40(3):277–9 [quiz E1-2].
13. Vaarala MH. Urinary Sample Collection Methods in Ileal Conduit Urinary Diversion Patients: A Randomized Control Trial. J Wound, Ostomy Cont Nurs 2018;45(1): 59–62.
14. Dolscheid-Pommerich RC, Klarmann-Schulz U, Conrad R, et al. Evaluation of the appropriate time period between sampling and analyzing for automated urinalysis. Biochem Med 2016;26(1):82–9.
15. Veljkovic K, Rodríguez-Capote K, Bhayana V, et al. Assessment of a four hour delay for urine samples stored without preservatives at room temperature for urinalysis. Clin Biochem 2012;45(10–11):856–8.
16. LaRocco MT, Franek J, Leibach EK, et al. Effectiveness of Preanalytic Practices on Contamination and Diagnostic Accuracy of Urine Cultures: a Laboratory Medicine Best Practices Systematic Review and Meta-analysis. Clin Microbiol Rev 2016;29(1):105–47.
17. Froom P, Bieganiec B, Ehrenrich Z, et al. Stability of common analytes in urine refrigerated for 24 h before automated analysis by test strips. Clin Chem 2000; 46(9):1384–6.

18. Simerville JA, Maxted WC, Pahira JJ. Urinalysis: a comprehensive review. Am Fam Physician 2005;71(6):1153–62.
19. Queremel Milani DA, Jialal I. Urinalysis. 2022. Treasure Island (FL): StatPearls; 2023.
20. Echeverry G, Hortin GL, Rai AJ. Introduction to urinalysis: historical perspectives and clinical application. Methods Mol Biol 2010;641:1–12.
21. Raymond JR, Yarger WE. Abnormal urine color: differential diagnosis. South Med J 1988;81(7):837–41.
22. Burg MD, Baerends EP, Hendrik Bell C. Unusual urine color during catheterization. Am Fam Physician 2016;94(7):572–4.
23. Cheng JT, Mohan S, Nasr SH, et al. Chyluria presenting as milky urine and nephrotic-range proteinuria. Kidney Int 2006;70(8):1518–22.
24. Saks M, Riviello R. Green urine discoloration in an otherwise healthy patient. Vis J Emerg Med 2015;1:12–3.
25. Blakey SA, Hixson-Wallace JA. Clinical significance of rare and benign side effects: propofol and green urine. Pharmacotherapy 2000;20(9):1120–2.
26. Ramírez-Guerrero G, Müller-Ortiz H, Pedreros-Rosales C. Polyuria in adults. a diagnostic approach based on pathophysiology. Rev Clin Esp 2022;222(5):301–8.
27. Bhasin B, Velez JCQ. Evaluation of polyuria: the roles of solute loading and water diuresis. Am J Kidney Dis 2016;67(3):507–11.
28. Chadha V, Garg U, Alon US. Measurement of urinary concentration: a critical appraisal of methodologies. Pediatr Nephrol 2001;16(4):374–82.
29. Proudfoot AT, Krenzelok EP, Vale JA. Position Paper on urine alkalinization. J Toxicol Clin Toxicol 2004;42(1):1–26.
30. Arnold MJ. Microscopic hematuria in adults: updated recommendations from the american urological association. Am Fam Physician 2021;104(6):655–7.
31. Abbate M, Zoja C, Remuzzi G. How does proteinuria cause progressive renal damage? J Am Soc Nephrol 2006;17(11):2974–84.
32. Haider M.Z., Aslam A., Proteinuria. 2022. In: StatPearls [Internet]. Treasure Island (FL): StatPearls Publishing; 2023.
33. Carroll MF, Temte JL. Proteinuria in adults: a diagnostic approach. Am Fam Physician 2000;62(6):1333–40.
34. Kidney Disease: Improving Global Outcomes (KDIGO) Glomerular Diseases Work Group. KDIGO 2021 Clinical practice guideline for the management of glomerular diseases. Kidney Int 2021;100(4S):S1–276.
35. White SL, Yu R, Craig JC, et al. Diagnostic accuracy of urine dipsticks for detection of albuminuria in the general community. Am J Kidney Dis 2011;58(1):19–28.
36. Snyder S, John JS. Workup for proteinuria. Prim Care 2014;41(4):719–35.
37. Rodby RA, Rohde RD, Sharon Z, et al. The urine protein to creatinine ratio as a predictor of 24-hour urine protein excretion in type 1 diabetic patients with nephropathy. The Collaborative Study Group. Am J Kidney Dis 1995;26(6):904–9.
38. Bellazreg F, Abid M, Lasfar NB, et al. Diagnostic value of dipstick test in adult symptomatic urinary tract infections: results of a cross-sectional Tunisian study. Pan Afr Med J 2019;33:131.
39. Perazella MA. The urine sediment as a biomarker of kidney disease. Am J Kidney Dis 2015;66(5):748–55.
40. Tsai JJ, Yeun JY, Kumar VA, et al. Comparison and interpretation of urinalysis performed by a nephrologist versus a hospital-based clinical laboratory. Am J Kidney Dis 2005;46(5):820–9.
41. Wise GJ, Schlegel PN. Sterile pyuria. N Engl J Med 2015;372(11):1048–54.

42. Muriithi AK, Nasr SH, Leung N. Utility of urine eosinophils in the diagnosis of acute interstitial nephritis. Clin J Am Soc Nephrol 2013;8(11):1857–62.
43. Nolan CR, Anger MS, Kelleher SP. Eosinophiluria–a new method of detection and definition of the clinical spectrum. N Engl J Med 1986;315(24):1516–9.
44. Muriithi AK, Leung N, Valeri AM, et al. Biopsy-proven acute interstitial nephritis, 1993-2011: a case series. Am J Kidney Dis 2014;64(4):558–66.
45. Köhler H, Wandel E, Brunck B. Acanthocyturia–a characteristic marker for glomerular bleeding. Kidney Int 1991;40(1):115–20.
46. Birch DF, Fairley KF. Haematuria: glomerular or non-glomerular? Lancet 1979; 2(8147):845–6.

Overview of, and Preparations for, Dialysis

Maryam Gondal, MD

KEYWORDS

- Chronic kidney disease stage 5 • Hemodialysis • Peritoneal dialysis
- Predialysis education • Renal replacement therapy

KEY POINTS

- Chronic kidney disease is a progressive condition with increase in incidence and prevalence due to enhanced longevity of general population.
- Chronic kidney disease stage 5 or end-stage renal disease is a major public health concern.
- Renal replacement therapy in the form of dialysis remains the main treatment for patients with kidney failure.
- Multidisciplinary patient education is the first step in preparing patients for dialysis and offering them support for selection of dialysis modality or conservative management.

INTRODUCTION

Chronic kidney disease (CKD) is a progressive condition which is defined by decreased kidney function evidenced by a glomerular filtration rate (GFR) less than 60 mL/min per 1.73 m^2 or markers of kidney damage, or both, for at least 3 months, regardless of the underlying cause.[1] CKD may be insidious, and most of the affected individuals remain asymptomatic. In most cases, kidney insufficiency is first noticed on routine laboratory work including urine studies. Signs and symptoms of CKD result from progressive uremia and other metabolic derangements, which, if left untreated, can inevitably lead to death. Based on international guidelines, CKD is classified into 5 stages (**Table 1**).

Renal replacement therapy (RRT) in the form of chronic dialysis or transplantation is the life-sustaining treatment for patients with kidney failure. The number of patients receiving dialysis is projected to steadily increase from 2.618 million in 2010 to 5.439 million in 2030 worldwide.[2] Because of the shortage of kidney donors and the comorbidities that develop with age, kidney transplantation is not always possible.[3] Dialysis remains the prevailing treatment option for most people with kidney failure.[4]

Department of Internal Medicine, Section of Nephrology, Yale School of Medicine, 330 Cedar Street, BB114, New Haven, CT 06510, USA
E-mail address: maryam.gondal@yale.edu

Med Clin N Am 107 (2023) 681–687
https://doi.org/10.1016/j.mcna.2023.03.003
0025-7125/23/© 2023 Elsevier Inc. All rights reserved.

Table 1
International guidelines for CKD

Stage	GFR (Description)	Range (mL/min/1.73 m^2)
1	Normal or high with structural or laboratory evidence of kidney disease	$\geq$90
2	Mild decrease in GFR	60–89
3a	Mild to moderate decrease in GFR	45–59
3b	Moderate decrease in GFR	30–44
4	Severe damage	15–29
5	End-stage kidney disease	<15

DISCUSSION

The term dialysis is derived from the Greek words dia, meaning "through", and lysis, meaning "loosening or splitting." The kidney's role of filtration of the blood is supplemented by artificial membranes and equipment, which remove excess water, solutes, and toxins. The apparatus needed to perform dialysis include a filter (also known as the dialyzer), dialysis solution (dialysate), and a machine to power the procedure. Dialysis can be intermittent or continuous. Continuous dialysis is reserved for hemodynamically unstable patients admitted to the intensive care unit. There are two types of intermittent dialysis procedures: hemodialysis (HD; using an external filter called dialyzer) or peritoneal dialysis (PD; using peritoneal membrane as the filter).

HD can be done in-center, where it is undertaken by support staff to aid in the dialytic procedure, or at home with proper training provided to the patients so that they can perform it themselves. It involves the removal of solutes across a semipermeable membrane down the concentration gradient by two mechanisms: diffusive clearance (random molecular motion) and convective clearance (osmotic force of water pushes solutes along with it through the membrane). The semipermeable membrane separates the blood from the dialysate which consists of highly purified water with sodium, potassium, magnesium, calcium, bicarbonate, chloride, and dextrose. During dialysis, a concentration equilibrium is prevented by continuous flowing of fresh dialysis solution in the dialyzer and replacing dialyzed blood with undialyzed blood. HD requires a high volume of ultrapure water to be used every treatment, which can be a challenge for city planners setting up dialysis units or patients doing dialysis at home.

To perform dialysis, the machine needs a blood flow of between 300 and 450 cc/min continuously. The specific type of vascular access chosen for HD is patient-centered, and there are three options available. These include arteriovenous fistula (AVF), arteriovenous graft (AVG), or a central venous catheter (CVC). AVF is the preferred access as it is associated with the lower rate of complications and has superior long-term durability. An AVF is created via a surgical anastomosis between an artery and a vein. Diversion of the high-flow arterial blood into the low-pressure vein results in progressive dilatation and wall thickening of the outflow vein, a process referred to as arterialization.[5] Arterialization eventually results in maturation, signifying the suitability of an AVF for cannulation regularly and HD.[5] An AVG is created by subcutaneously tunneling an expanded polytetrafluoroethylene graft, connecting an inflow artery and an outflow vein via a surgical anastomosis. AVGs are more prone to infection and thrombosis than AVFs, and they are therefore usually considered only when AVF options have been exhausted.[6] CVCs are used in patients requiring urgent HD who may be awaiting permanent access creation, access maturation, or kidney transplantation.[5] They are also used as permanent HD access in patients who have exhausted their AVF or AVG options. CVCs have many advantages, including a less-demanding technical procedure (typically inserted by radiologists, nephrologists, and intensivists, rather than surgeons), lower resource usage, potential for immediate HD provision, and no need for percutaneous cannulation (unlike AVFs and AVGs). This makes them a convenient, albeit inferior, form of vascular access. They are not the optimal choice because they have a high risk of infection, they malfunction frequently, and they thrombose. Catheters come in two varieties: nontunneled catheters (used in patients who are critically ill for short duration) and tunneled catheters (long-term use).

In PD, fluid (dialysate) is instilled in the peritoneal cavity, and solutes diffuse from the blood in the peritoneal capillaries into the dialysate, effecting an exchange analogous to that of HD. Similarly, imposition of a transcapillary osmotic gradient creates the driving force for ultrafiltration of fluid from the capillaries into the dialysate. In contrast to HD, in which the pressure that is applied is hydrostatic, PD involves osmotic pressure created by the intraperitoneal instillation of hypertonic dialysate, usually as glucose in the form of 1.5%, 2.5%, or 4.25% dextrose. Higher concentrations of glucose exert higher osmotic pressures and effect greater degrees of ultrafiltration. To access the peritoneal cavity, a single-lumen, silicone rubber Tenckhoff catheter (Medtronic) traversing the anterior abdominal wall is used. The catheter is positioned with the tip in the true pelvis. The catheter then passes through the rectus abdominis muscle, to which it is anchored by a Dacron cuff, and is then tunneled subcutaneously to the exit site, where it leaves the body.

PD may be performed manually, usually three or four times daily, with the dialysate dwelling in the abdominal cavity between exchanges to equilibrate; this is termed continuous ambulatory peritoneal dialysis (CAPD). Alternatively, a machine, commonly referred to as a "cycler," may be used to perform a number of exchanges overnight in a procedure called automated peritoneal dialysis (APD). These patients will perform all their dialysis processes overnight when they are sleeping so that their days are free. The type of dialysis chosen for a patient, CAPD versus APD, depends on patient preferences, local resources, and infrastructure.

PREPARATION FOR DIALYSIS

Preparation for RRT should begin early enough in the course of CKD to allow time for patients to consider different treatment options and to establish a permanent functioning access for the dialysis modality of choice. In determining how early to begin the preparation of patients for dialysis, it is useful to consider that it can take 1 to 3 months of interactive CKD education for patients to accept potential need for RRT and to decide which therapy best meets their expectations and fits their lifestyle. Early patient education for those with CKD is shown to be highly effective when focused on health promotion, shared decision-making, and discussion of treatment options.[7] In 1 randomized, controlled trial on patient education, a one-on-one educational session followed by phone calls every 3 weeks significantly extended the time to requiring dialysis.[7] Post hoc analyses from this clinical trial, as well as findings from other observational studies, demonstrate a variety of additional benefits from patient education: reduced patient anxiety; delay in dialysis need; reduced number of hospitalizations; reduced numbers of emergency room and physician visits; increased likelihood that the patient will remain employed in work and be more adherent to therapy; and reduced mortality.[8]

Sufficient time also needs to be allocated for placement and maturation of dialysis access. The mean time for AVF maturation is 3 months. AVGs can be ready in about 2 weeks. Moreover, a substantial proportion of new fistulae/grafts fail to achieve suitability for dialysis treatment; therefore, the first vascular access should be placed sufficiently early to allow enough time to either revise the initial access or for a second access to be placed and mature prior to the initiation of dialysis.[9] Vascular catheters are an option but pose higher risks of infections and are used as a last resort for long-term dialysis. PD catheters need to be placed at least 2 weeks in advance to prevent leak.

The Kidney Disease Improving Global Outcomes Clinical Practice Guidelines recommend initiating dialysis when there are symptoms or signs that are indicative of kidney failure (eg, lethargy, change in taste, fatigue, acid-base or electrolyte abnormalities, or pruritus) rather than basing it off any individual creatinine. Some of the other symptoms encouraging initiation are the inability to control volume status or blood pressure, progressive deterioration in nutritional status refractory to dietary intervention, or development of cognitive impairment.[10] A specific estimated glomerular filtration rate (eGFR) value for initiating dialysis in the absence of symptomatic kidney failure has not been established. The Initiating Dialysis Early and Late study did not demonstrate any clinical benefit in commencing dialysis at higher levels of eGFR, and the variability in measurement of eGFR in CKD stage 5 is such that it should not be considered to reliably reflect kidney function.[11] There is no reason to start dialysis in anticipation of these symptoms.

MANAGING STAGE 5 CKD IN THE ELDERLY

Patients aged 70 years or older constitute the fastest-growing segment of the dialysis population.[12] The option of a conservative approach to the management of older patients with advanced CKD as an alternative to dialysis therapy has generated increased interest in clinical practice, particularly as end-stage kidney disease has increasingly become a geriatric-associated condition.[12] Older adults have an increased burden of comorbidities and geriatric problems, including cognitive decline and frailty. Initiation of dialysis can adversely affect the quality of life because of difficulties in transportation, changes in lifestyle, and loss of independence.[13] Patients with more comorbidities consistently die earlier on dialysis and do not have a demonstrable survival benefit from dialysis compared to those who are treated conservatively.[14] A maximum conservative management strategy for the elderly and those with multiple comorbid conditions and advanced CKD has been proposed, especially in Europe.[15] Programs that encourage a conservative approach call for comprehensive care with multidisciplinary teams including dieticians, social workers, nurses, and physicians. Patients receive intensive management of complications of CKD, which include anemia, mineral bone disease, volume management, and electrolytes disturbances. Special attention is paid to advance care planning discussions with patients who have limited life expectancy and early designation of legal guardian before the onset of cognitive impairment is encouraged.[16] Primary care providers play a critical role in these discussions as they often have a longitudinal relationship with the patient and their family that can be very meaningful and provide great insight into this decision.

DISORDERS ASSOCIATED WITH STAGE 5 CKD
Mineral and Bone Disorders

Disorders of mineral and bone metabolism are common in patients with stage 5 CKD and are associated with increase in cardiovascular calcification, contributing to increase risk of complications and death.[17] There is decreased renal phosphate excretion and decreased conversion of vitamin D to its active form, 1,25-dihydroxyvitamin D, which results in reduction in absorption of intestinal calcium. The hyperphosphatemia, hypocalcemia, and decreased levels of active vitamin D cause an increase in synthesis and secretion of parathyroid hormone. Hyperparathyroidism is independently associated with increased mortality and higher prevalence of cardiovascular disease.[18] Current guidelines recommend monitoring calcium and phosphate levels (every 3–4 months), parathyroid hormone levels (every 6–12 months), and bone-specific alkaline phosphatase activity (every 6–12 months).[17] Patients with persistent high levels of parathyroid hormone should restrict dietary phosphate intake. If phosphate levels are not controlled with dietary restriction, then phosphate binder such as Renvela (sevelamer carbonate), Velphoro (sucroferric oxyhydroxide), Auryxia (ferric citrate), Fosrenol (lanthanum carbonate), or Phoslo (calcium acetate) is prescribed with meals. Serum levels of 25-OH vitamin D are also decreased in patient with stage 5 CKD, and supplementation is recommended if levels fall below 30 ng/mL.

Anemia

Anemia is common in patients with stage 5 CKD because of deficient erythropoietin synthesis, iron deficiency, blood loss, and decreased erythrocyte half-life.[19] The use of erythropoiesis-stimulating agents results in a reduced need for blood transfusions and also has been associated with a reduction in left ventricular hypertrophy.[20] Iron status should be carefully assessed to ensure that transferrin saturation is between 20% and 50% and ferritin levels are between 100 and 800 ng/mL.[19] Supplementation can be achieved with either oral or parenteral iron administration early in CKD stages, but by the time patients are on dialysis, parenteral iron is recommended.

Electrolyte and Acid-Base Disturbances

Hyperkalemia can develop in stage 5 CKD patients due to impaired GFR and high dietary potassium intake along with the use of renin-angiotensin aldosterone system blockers that inhibit renal potassium excretion. If potassium levels are below 5.5 mmol/L, patients can be managed with dietary changes with the expertise of a renal dietician. Higher levels warrant the use of potassium binders like Kayexalate (sodium polystyrene sulfonate), Veltassa (patiromer), or Lokelma (sodium zirconium cyclosilicate), which can be prescribed chronically to stave off dialysis initiation.

A non-anion-gap metabolic acidosis can develop in patients with CKD, primarily owing to reduction in renal ammonia synthesis and titratable acid (phosphate) excretion. Retention of organic acids due to uremia can lead to increased anion-gap metabolic acidosis in patients with stage 5 CKD. Acidosis adversely affects bone mineral content and promotes skeletal muscle catabolism. Current guidelines recommend treating metabolic acidosis with alkali therapy if serum bicarbonate concentration is <22 mEq/L. In a randomized trial, oral sodium bicarbonate supplementation slowed the progression of CKD.[21] Bicarbonate supplementation can be given as a prescribed tablet or in the form of common baking soda mixed with water if cost is an issue.

SUMMARY

CKD is a progressive condition with associated morbidity and mortality. The global incidence of kidney failure is rising, and dialysis remains the main treatment for majority of the patients. Dialysis modality decision-making is a complex process, influenced by patient's health literacy, willingness to accept information, predialysis lifestyle, comorbid conditions, support systems and values.

CLINICS CARE POINTS

- Renal replacement therapy in the form of dialysis or kidney transplant is the life-sustaining treatment for patients with kidney failure.

- Kidney transplant is not possible for all patients because of shortage of organs and comorbidities in some patients which would prevent them from benefitting from the surgery.

- Dialysis is the main treatment option for most patients with advanced kidney failure.

- Multidisciplinary patient education is the first step in preparing patients for dialysis and offering them support for selection of dialysis modality or conservative management.

- The decision to start dialysis is individualized and is based on appearance of symptoms rather than a specific number of creatinine or eGFR.

DISCLOSURE

The authors have nothing to disclose.

REFERENCES

1. Webster AC, Nagler EV, Morton RL, et al. Chronic kidney disease. Lancet 2017; 389:1238–52.
2. Liyanage T, Ninomiya T, Jha V, et al. Worldwide access to treatment for end-stage kidney disease: a systematic review. Lancet 2015;385(9981):1975–82.
3. Song MK. Quality of life of patients with advanced chronic kidney disease receiving conservative care without dialysis. Semin Dial 2016;29:165–9.
4. Bello AK, Levin A, Lunney M, et al. Status of care for end stage kidney disease in countries and regions worldwide: international cross sectional survey. BMJ 2019; 367:l5873.
5. Lok CE, Huber TS, Lee T, et al. KDOQI clinical practice guideline for vascular access: 2019 update. Am J Kidney Dis 2020;75(4 Suppl 2):S1–164 [Erratum in: Am J Kidney Dis, 2021;77(4):551].
6. Murad MH, Elamin MB, Sidawy AN, et al. Autogenous versus prosthetic vascular access for hemodialysis: a systematic review and meta-analysis. J Vasc Surg 2008;48(5 Suppl):34S–47S.
7. Hain D, Calvin DJ, Simmons DE Jr. CKD education: an evolving concept. Nephrol Nurs J 2009;36:317–9.
8. Devins GM, Mendelssohn DC, Barre PE, et al. Predialysis psychoeducational intervention and coping styles influence time to dialysis in chronic kidney disease. Am J Kidney Dis 2003;42:693–703.
9. Coresh J, Walser M, Hill S. Survival on dialysis among chronic renal failure patients treated with a supplemented low-protein diet before dialysis. J Am Soc Nephrol 1995;6:1379–85.
10. Kidney Disease Improving Global Outcomes (KDIGO) Work Group. KDIGO 2012 clinical practice guideline for the evaluation and management of chronic kidney disease. Kidney Int Suppl 2013;3:1–150.
11. Wong MG, Pollock CA, Cooper BA, et al. Association between GFR estimated by multiple methods at dialysis commencement and patient survival. Clin J Am Soc Nephrol 2014;9:135–42.

12. United States Renal Data System. 2014 USRDS annual data report: epidemiology of kidney disease in the United States. Bethesda: National Institutes of Health; 2014.
13. Berger JR, Hedayati SS. Renal replacement therapy in the elderly population. Clin J Am Soc Nephrol 2012;7:1039–46.
14. Couchoud C, Labeeuw M, Moranne O, et al. A clinical score to predict 6-month prognosis in elderly patients starting dialysis for end-stage renal disease. Nephrol Dial Transplant 2009;24:1553–61.
15. Carson RC, Juszczak M, Davenport A, et al. Is maximum conservative management an equivalent treatment option to dialysis for elderly patients with significant comorbid disease? Clin J Am Soc Nephrol 2009;4:1611–9.
16. Grubbs V, Moss AH, Cohen LM, et al. A palliative approach to dialysis care: a patient-centered transition to the end of life. Clin J Am Soc Nephrol 2014;9: 2203–9.
17. Kidney Disease: Improving Global Outcomes (KDIGO) CKD-MBD Working Group. KDIGO clinical practice guideline for diagnosis, evaluation, prevention, and treatment of chronic kidney disease-mineral and bone disorder (CKD-MBD). Kidney Int Suppl 2009;113:S1–130.
18. Kestenbaum B, Sampson JN, Rudser KD, et al. Serum phosphate levels and mortality risk among people with chronic kidney disease. J Am Soc Nephrol 2005;16: 520–8.
19. KDOQIKDOQI clinical practice guideline and clinical practice recommendations for anemia in chronic kidney disease: 2007 update of hemoglobin target. Am J Kidney Dis 2007;50:471–530.
20. Parfrey PS, Lauve M, Latremouille-Viau D, et al. Erythropoietin therapy and left ventricular mass index in CKD and ESRD patients: a meta-analysis. Clin J Am Soc Nephrol 2009;4:755–76.
21. De Brito-Ashurst I, Varagunam M, Raftery MJ, et al. Bicarbonate supplementation slows progression of CKD and improves nutritional status. J Am Soc Nephrol 2009;20:2075–84.

Diabetic Kidney Disease
An Update

Sonali Gupta, MD*, Mary Dominguez, MD,
Ladan Golestaneh, MD, MS

KEYWORDS

- Diabetic kidney disease • Diabetic nephropathy • Albuminuria • Proteinuria
- Chronic kidney disease • End-stage kidney disease

KEY POINTS

- Diabetic kidney disease (DKD) is the leading cause of chronic kidney disease and end-stage kidney disease in the United States and worldwide.
- DKD is asymptomatic in early stages and routine screening is necessary for an early diagnosis.
- The most effective interventions remain lifestyle changes aimed at smoking cessation, reduction of obesity, hypertension, and hyperglycemia.
- All patients with DKD should be treated with an angiotensin-converting enzyme inhibitor or angiotensin II receptor blocker as tolerated. Among the anti-hyperglycemic agents, first-line treatment remains, metformin (renally dosed) and sodium-glucose co-transporter-2 inhibitors. Glucagon-like peptide-1 receptor agonists and non-steroidal mineralocorticoid receptor antagonists should be considered for add-on therapy.

INTRODUCTION

Diabetes is a major public health challenge in both developed and developing countries. It is estimated that in 2030, 643 million people will be living with diabetes.[1] About 1 in 10 Americans have diabetes, and 1 in 3 American adults have prediabetes.[2] Up to 35% of patients with diabetes develop kidney disease.[3] The increased incidence of diabetes in some populations may also be related to intra-uterine events, epigenetic risks, and adverse social determinants of health.[4,5] Thus, the diabetes epidemic will increasingly affect the most vulnerable individuals in future generations. Recent large clinical trials testing the efficacy of pharmaceuticals in improving diabetes outcomes introduce a glimmer of hope for containing this epidemic.

This review describes the epidemiology, pathogenesis, and diagnosis of diabetic kidney disease (DKD) and focuses on evidence-based management for DKD including

Department of Medicine, Division of Nephrology, Albert Einstein College of Medicine, 3411 Wayne Avenue, 5th Floor, Bronx, NY 10467, USA
* Corresponding author.
E-mail address: sogupta@montefiore.org

Med Clin N Am 107 (2023) 689–705
https://doi.org/10.1016/j.mcna.2023.03.004
0025-7125/23/© 2023 Elsevier Inc. All rights reserved.

control of hyperglycemia, hypertension, hyperlipidemia, and albuminuria with emerging pharmaceutical options.

TERMINOLOGY

Diabetic nephropathy (DN) is a common long-term complication of Type 1 and Type 2 diabetes. DKD, a more encompassing diagnostic term than DN, is the leading cause of chronic kidney disease (CKD) and end-stage kidney disease (ESKD) requiring dialysis or transplantation in the United States and worldwide.[1,6,7] DN manifests as albuminuria and progressive renal failure, while other non-DN categories of DKD include atherosclerosis of the renal arteries, renal arteriolosclerosis, and acute kidney injury episodes related to heart disease, and are not characterized by albuminuria.[8]

PREVALENCE

Approximately 30% to 40% of individuals with diabetes develop DN, during their lifetime.[9] The epidemiology of DKD is changing with prevalence quickly outpacing incidence as diabetes increasingly affects younger individuals with fewer comorbidities and longer lifespan. Improvements in cardiovascular survival related to novel therapeutics also increase the prevalence of DKD.[10]

COST

The cost burden of DKD and ESKD is enormous.[11] Comorbidities including stroke, heart disease, and hypertension result in cumulative accrual of cost because of the need for hospitalizations, ambulatory care, pharmaceuticals, and cardiovascular interventions.[12] Progression through CKD stages is closely associated with a synergistic increase in cost.[11] Early recognition of DKD and aggressive risk factor mitigation can reduce this cost burden.[13] Despite clear screening guidelines by the American Diabetes Association (ADA) advocating for urinary albumin to creatinine ratios (UACR) and estimated glomerular filtration rate (eGFR) measurements at least annually[14]; DKD is underdiagnosed in early stages which presents a challenge to risk mitigation efforts.

RISK FACTORS

Older age, Black race, and Hispanic ethnicity,[15] genetic predisposition as demonstrated in alarmingly high rates of disease among Pima Indians[16] and Alaska natives,[17] and male sex, all demonstrate a high proclivity toward diabetes and DKD.[1] Patients with a longer duration of diabetes and uncontrolled status are also at high risk, especially in the presence of other manifestations of microvascular organ damage.[18] Obesity is an independent risk factor for the development and progression of DKD.[19]

PATHOGENESIS OF DIABETIC KIDNEY DISEASE

The pathogenesis of progressive DKD is driven by an interplay of metabolic derangements, hemodynamic alterations, and immune dysregulation.[20,21] DKD is classified into (1) the classical albuminuric phenotype with histological features of diabetic glomerulopathy (DN); and (2) the non-albuminuric phenotype, characterized by predominant vascular lesions and/or tubulointerstitial fibrosis with relatively intact glomerular structure.[22,23] The predominant glomerular lesions in DN are characterized by thickened glomerular basement membrane, mesangial expansion, and podocyte injury in early stages, followed by diffuse glomerulosclerosis, arteriolar hyalinosis, tubulointerstitial fibrosis, and atrophy in later stages. On electron microscopy, there is foot process effacement, podocyte detachment, reduction, and atrophy.[24] Persistently elevated blood glucose levels result in accumulation of advanced glycated end-products (AGE) precursors which activate the protein C and aldose reductase pathway, both of which are responsible for generation of reactive oxygen species and accelerate glomerular and tubular apoptosis and vascular pathology in diabetes.[25–27] AGEs also induce epithelial to mesenchymal cell transformation in podocytes leading to fibrosis and scarring.[28]

Non-albuminuric DKD is characterized by predominant atherosclerosis, atypical vascular lesions, and/or tubulointerstitial fibrosis instead of podocyte injury.[29] Hemodynamic disturbances play an important role in the pathogenesis and include aberrant activation of various vasoactive hormone pathways including renin-angiotensin-aldosterone system (RAAS) and endothelin.[30] These hemodynamic alterations activate intracellular second messengers and growth factors, which in turn, result in systemic and glomerular hypertension.[31]

DIAGNOSIS OF DIABETIC KIDNEY DISEASE

DN is characterized clinically by the presence of persistent albuminuria and/or reduced renal function demonstrated on two measurements with at least a 3-month difference in the timing of measurements.[15,32] DN is dependent on demonstrating urinary albumin amount >30 mg/24 hours which is diagnosed on a 24-hour urine collection or a spot UACR, with risk of progression closely associated with degree of albuminuria. Albuminuria less than 30 mg is known as mild, with albuminuria >30 mg and <300 mg as moderate and >300 mg as severe albuminuria. (**Fig. 1**).[33] Low eGFR in the absence of albuminuria is the other diagnostic marker for DKD and is an important prognostic marker for cardiovascular outcomes irrespective of albuminuria.[34]

SCREENING FOR DIABETIC KIDNEY DISEASE

DKD is asymptomatic in early stages and routine screening is necessary for an early diagnosis. The 2022 ADA Standards of Medical Care in Diabetes and the 2022 Kidney Disease: Improving Global Outcomes (KDIGO) Clinical Practice Guidelines recommend routine annual screening of diabetic patients for kidney disease by checking eGFR and UACR.[35,36] For Type 1 diabetes, CKD screening starts at 5 years after diagnosis of diabetes. For Type 2 diabetes, screening should start at the time of diabetes diagnosis. Renal function is routinely reported by eGFR using the Chronic Kidney Disease Epidemiology Collaboration (CKD-EPI) equation. In 2021, The American Society of Nephrology (ASN) and National Kidney Foundation (NKF) advocated the removal of the race modifier in CKD-EPI equation for calculating renal function.[37] Primary care physicians should consider referring patients with eGFR <60 mL/min/1.73 m^2 and moderately elevated albuminuria to nephrologists. All patients should be referred to a nephrologist once there is severe albuminuria or when eGFR drops below 45 mL/min/1.73 m^2 (see **Fig. 1**).

DIABETIC KIDNEY DISEASE TREATMENT

There is no cure for DKD and regression of adverse pathophysiological changes once they start, occurs very infrequently[38] (**Fig. 2**). Broadly speaking, the management of DKD is directed toward delaying progression of kidney disease and preventing cardiovascular complications. Albuminuria reduction, glycemic control, and blood pressure control comprise surrogate endpoints that can be targeted to delay progression of kidney disease. Recent development in pharmaceuticals offer hope in curbing the

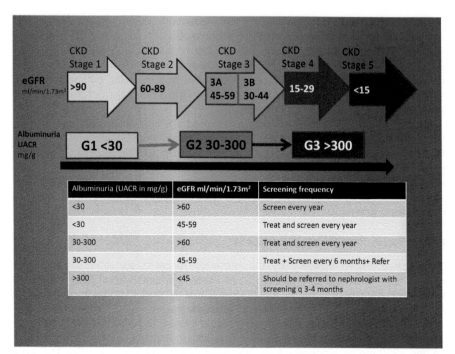

Fig. 1. Risk categories of CKD based on eGFR and albuminuria and screening frequency in these stages. eGFR, estimated glomerular filtration rate; UACR, urine albumin creatinine ratio.

incidence and progression of DKD.[39] Most of these therapeutics have proven extremely effective in clinical studies but challenges remain in successful implementation.[40] The most effective interventions involve lifestyle changes such as reducing smoking, obesity, hypertension, and hyperglycemia.[36,41]

LIFESTYLE MODIFICATION

Lifestyle modification should be the initial intervention in the management of DKD. Dietary modifications include (1) low salt diet and (2) low protein diet. A low salt diet is recommended for control of blood pressure, for reducing proteinuria,[42] and for enhancing the antiproteinuric and blood pressure-reducing benefits of RAAS inhibitors (RAASi).[43] Multiple guidelines including KDIGO 2022 suggest targeting a sodium intake <2 g of sodium per day (or <90 mmol of sodium per day, or <5 g of sodium chloride per day) in patients with hypertension and CKD.[36,44–46] Dietary protein restriction has been extensively studied and shown to reduce progression of CKD in later stages.[47–49] The National Kidney Foundation Kidney Disease Outcomes Quality Initiative (NKF-KDOQI) recommends a protein consumption of 0.6 to 0.8 g/kg/day for patients with diabetes and CKD.[50] However very low protein diets can lead to malnutrition and deficiency of important amino acids. The ADA and KDIGO recommended that medical professionals and patients work as a team to optimize nutrition, weight, exercise, and smoking cessation.[36,44]

BLOOD PRESSURE CONTROL

Numerous trials have shown that blood pressure control can reduce proteinuria and is associated with better cardiovascular outcomes in DKD. RAASi (angiotensin-

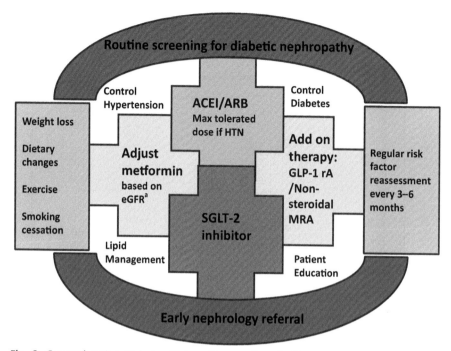

Fig. 2. Comprehensive Diabetes Kidney Disease Care. [a]eGFR 30 to 45 mL/min/1.73 m2: reduce dose of metformin, eGFR <30 mL/min/1.73 m2: stop metformin, ACEI, angiotensin-converting enzyme inhibitor; ARB, angiotensin receptor blocker; DN, diabetic nephrology; GLP-1 RA, glucagon-like peptide 1 receptor agonist; MRA, mineralocorticoid receptor antagonist; SGLT-2 inhibitor, sodium glucose co-transporter 2 inhibitor.

converting enzyme inhibitor [ACEi] or angiotensin receptor blockers [ARBs]) are the preferred choice for antihypertensive medications for patients with DKD, especially those with evidence of albuminuria. Blood pressure goals for patients with DKD may differ depending on the task force or organization from which recommendations are taken. The ADA and American College of Cardiology/American Heart Association task force recommended a BP target of < 130/80 mm Hg.[51,52] KDIGO suggests treating adults with hypertension and DKD to a target systolic blood pressure of <120 mm Hg.[44] The African American Study of Kidney Disease and Hypertension (AASK trial) showed that tighter blood pressure control with mean arterial pressure goal of ≤92 versus 102 to 107 mm Hg was associated with more significant reduction in proteinuria, however tight control blood pressure was complicated by hypotension and AKI.[53] Thus, a tailored approach is necessary for each patient.

GLYCEMIC CONTROL

Population studies have shown that glycemic control leads to a significant reduction in microvascular complications in patients with diabetes (**Table 1**).[18] The United Kingdom Prospective Diabetes Study (UKPDS 33, 1998), the Epidemiology of Diabetes Interventions and Complications (EDIC, 2004) trial, Action to Control Cardiovascular Risk in Diabetes (ACCORD, 2008), Action in Diabetes and Vascular Disease: Preterax and Diamicron Modified Release Controlled Evaluation (ADVANCE, 2008) trial, and the Veterans Affairs Diabetes Trial (VADT, 2009) contributed crucial data to

Table 1
Major epidemiological trials studying effect of intensive glucose control on macrovascular and microvascular complications associated with diabetes

Clinical Trial Name	Type of Diabetes	Mean Duration of Diabetes	Hgb1ac	Macrovascular Complications	Microvascular Complications	Adverse Events in Intensive Group	Follow-up Period
UKPDS	T2DM	Newly diagnosed	Intensive glycemic control (fasting glucose <108 mg/dL). Median Hb1ac 7.0% vs 7.9%	Non-significant trend toward decreased myocardial infarction.	Significant reduction in microvascular endpoint, particularly retinopathy requiring photocoagulation	Increased weight gain and hypoglycemia, particularly in patients treated with insulin	10 y
DCCT	T1DM	1–15 y	Goal Hb1ac <6.05%	No CV benefits	Improvement in microalbuminuria, retinopathy, and neuropathy	Increased risk of hypoglycemia	6.5 y (range 3–9 y)
Follow-up of DCCT: EDIC				Intensive diabetes therapy during the DCCT (6.5 y) has persistent long-term cardiovascular benefit that persists for up to 30 y	Persistent improved microvascular endpoints		30 y
ACCORD	T2DM	10 y	Target HbA1c <6% vs standard glycemic control targeting a HbA1c 7%–7.9%	No CV benefits	N/A	Increased all-cause and CV mortality	3.4 y
ADVANCE	T2DM	8 y	Target HbA1c ≤ 6.5%	No reduction in the risk of macrovascular events	23% reduction in the risk of microvascular events, mainly nephropathy	Increased risk of severe hypoglycemia and an increased rate of hospitalization	5 y

VADT	T2DM	11.5 y	Intensive group. If HbA1c >6%, insulin added At 5.6 y of follow-up, intensive vs standard Hb1ac was 6.9% vs 8.4%	No CV benefits 11.5 VADT follow-up after 10 y: Showed significant CV benefit in intensive therapy. 8.6 major cardiovascular events prevented per 1000 person-years	No difference in incidence or progression of retinopathy, nephropathy, or neuropathy	More frequent hypoglycemia	6 y

Abbreviations: ACCORD, the action to control cardiovascular risk in diabetes trial; ADVANCE, action in diabetes and vascular disease, Preterax and Diamicron Modified Release Controlled Evaluation; CV, cardiovascular; DCCT, diabetes control and complications trial; DM, diabetes mellitus; EDIC, the Epidemiology of Diabetes Interventions and Complications trial; Hgb A1c, hemoglobin A1c; UKPDS 33, The United Kingdom Prospective Diabetes Study; VADT, the Veterans Affairs Diabetes Trial.

build consensus guidelines.[54–58] One of the earliest and largest randomized controlled trials, UKPDS, showed that intensive glycemic control resulted in a trend toward reduction of cardiovascular risk in patients with newly diagnosed diabetes in the initial study period, followed by a significant reduction in the incidence of microvascular complication, and death from any cause at 10 years follow-up.[59] Similarly, although the initial Diabetes Control and Complications Trial (DCCT, 1993) did not show a significant effect of intensive glycemic control in Type 1 diabetes on cardiovascular events, the the follow-up EDIC trial did show delayed renal decline and significant benefit on cardiovascular outcomes.[58,60] Intensive glycemic control must be balanced with the risk of hypoglycemia in those with comorbidities, as it is associated with increased cardiovascular events and mortality.[61]

RECOMMENDED ANTI-HYPERGLYCEMIC MEDICATIONS

Metformin remains the cornerstone of drug management in patients with diabetes. UKPDS reported lower cardiovascular mortality and morbidity in patients treated with metformin in comparison with alternative glucose-lowering drugs, despite similar glycemic control.[62] Metformin is not recommended for eGFR< 30 (26) and should be discontinued to prevent serious complications of lactic acidosis.[63]

Sodium Glucose Co-Transported inhibitors 2 (SGLT2i) are medications that reduce the risk of ESKD, or death due to kidney disease in people with type 2 diabetes.[64] This class of medication blocks glucose absorption at the S1 segment of the proximal convoluted tubule which reabsorbs 90% of the glucose filtered by the glomerulus. This leads to glycosuria and achieves glycemic control.[65–68] The primary mechanism by which SGLT2 inhibitors are nephroprotective, however, is through the increase of distal sodium delivery and increased of tubule-glomerular feedback resulting in afferent vasoconstriction and reduction in intraglomerular pressure (**Fig. 3**).[69] Other potential mechanisms of action by which SGLT2s work include improved cardiac function, decreased tubular transport burden associated with decrease in oxygen consumption and oxidative stress.[70] A detailed review of the clinical trials testing SGLT2i is presented in **Table 2**. Dapagliflozin was approved by the FDA on 30 April, 2022, to reduce the risk of kidney function decline, kidney failure, cardiovascular death, and hospitalization for heart failure in adults with CKD (35). These medications

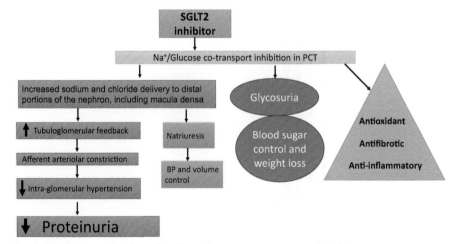

Fig. 3. Mechanism of action of sodium glucose co-transporter-2 inhibitors.

Table 2
Major landmark trials on treatment of diabetic kidney disease

Trial Name	Diabetes Type and Target Population	N	Intervention	Outcomes
ROADMAP	T2DM without microalbuminuria	4449	Olmesartan vs placebo	Olmesartan delayed the onset of microalbuminuria
IRMA-2	T2DM and microalbuminuria	590	Irbesartan 150 mg vs Irbesartan 300 mg vs Placebo	Irbesartan reduced development of overt proteinuria
Captopril- trial	T1DM with proteinuria	409	Captopril 25 mg 3x/day vs placebo	Captopril reduced the risk for doubling of SCr as a primary outcome and death, dialysis and transplant as secondary outcome
IDNT	T2DM with proteinuria and reduced kidney function	1715	Irbesartan vs amlodipine vs placebo	Irbesartan reduced the risk for doubling of SCr, ESKD, or death
RENAAL	T2DM with proteinuria and reduced kidney function	1513	Losartan vs Placebo	Losartan reduced the risk for doubling of SCr, ESKD, or death
CREDENCE	T2DM, CKD with eGFR >30–<90 and albuminuria of 0.3–5 gr	4401	Canagliflozin 100 mg vs placebo. All patients were on RAASi	The risk of kidney failure and cardiovascular events was 30% lower in the canagliflozin group than in the placebo
DAPA-CKD	Patients with and with or without Type 2DM, with CKD with eGFR 25–75 and albuminuria o 0.2–5 gr	4304	Dapagliflozin 10 mg vs placebo. Most of the patients on RAASi	The risk for CKD progression, and death from renal or cardiovascular causes was significantly lower in the treatment group when compared with the placebo group
EMPA-REG	Patients with CKD with eGFR of 20 to <45 or eGFR of 45 to <90 and 200 mg of albuminuria. With or without T2DM	6609	Empagliflozin 10 mg vs placebo	Treatment group had lower risk of progression of kidney disease or death from cardiovascular causes than placebo

(continued on next page)

Table 2
(continued)

Trial Name	Diabetes Type and Target Population	N	Intervention	Outcomes
FIDELIO-DKD	CKD with eGFR 25 to <75, albuminuria and T2DM	5734	Finerenone 10 mg (eGFR<60 60 mL/min/1.73 m²) or 20 mg (eGFR>60 mL/min/1.73 m²) vs placebo. 98.8% on RAASi	Finerenone reduced the risk for DKD progression and cardiovascular events as compared to placebo in patients with DKD
FIGARO-DKD	CKD2-4, albuminuria and T2DM	7437	Finerenone 10 mg (eGFR<60) or 20 mg (eGFR>60 mL/min/1.73 m²) vs placebo	Finerenone therapy improved cardiovascular outcomes as compared with placebo in patients with DM, CKD, and albuminuria

Abbreviations: CKD, chronic kidney disease; CREDENCE, canagliflozin and renal events in diabetes and nephropathy clinical evaluation; DAPA-CKD, the dapagliflozin in chronic kidney disease trial; DM; diabetes mellitus; eGFR, estimated glomerular filtration rate; EMPA-KIDNEY, the empagliflozin, cardiovascular outcome, and mortality in type 2 diabetes mellitus; ESKD, end-stage kidney disease; FIDELIO-CKD, Effect of Finerenone on Chronic Kidney Disease Outcomes in Type 2 diabetes; FIGARO-DKD, Cardiovascular Events with Finerenone in Kidney Disease and Type 2 DiabetesIDNT, the irbesartan diabetic nephropathy trial; IRMA-2, Irbesartan in Patients with Type 2 Diabetes and Microalbuminuria trial; RAASi, renin-angiotensin-aldosterone inhibitor; RENAAL, The Reduction of Endpoints in NIDDM with the angiotensin II antagonist losartan trial; ROADMAP, the randomized olmesartan and diabetes microalbuminuria prevention; SCr, serum creatinine.

are strongly recommended by KDIGO and ADA for the management of DKD and albu-minuria.[44,45] A small decrease in eGFR can be expected when these medications are initiated but this decrease is followed by stabilization of GFR and a slower decline in renal function.[71] Because of glycosuria, SGLT2is are also associated with a two-to-four-fold increased risk of genitourinary infections[71,72] and patients should be educated to monitor for any evidence of genital irritation or discharge and to maintain genital hygiene.

Glucagon-like peptide 1 agonists (GLP-1a) are effective in glycemic control, and as an added benefit, induce weight loss. GLP-1as have shown cardiovascular benefits by reducing all cardiovascular outcomes[73–75] and have also proven to reduce onset of microalbuminuria and slow eGFR decline in patients with diabetes.[35,76,77] KDIGO recommends addition of GLP1a in patients already on metformin and SGLT2i that have not achieved glycemic control goal.[44]

OTHER DIABETIC KIDNEY DISEASE AND DIABETIC NEPHROPATHY PROTECTIVE MEDICATIONS
Renin-Angiotensin-Aldosterone System Inhibitors Medications

Activation of the renin-angiotensin system has an important role in the development and pathogenesis of DN. There is abundant evidence to support the benefits of RAAS inhibition with ACE inhibitors and ARBs in proteinuria reduction, blood pressure control, and decreasing progression of kidney disease (see **Table 2**).[78–83] These reno-protective benefits are independent of blood pressure control.[81] It is recommended to monitor serum creatinine and potassium levels after initiation or after increasing the dose of these medications.

Lipid Lowering Medications

Because dyslipidemia is a major cardiovascular risk factor in patients with type 2 diabetes, lipid-lowering agents are another important therapy for patients with DKD.[84] The Study of Heart and Renal Protection trial aimed to assess the safety and efficacy of reducing low density lipoprotein (LDL) cholesterol in more than 9000 patients with CKD and showed that simvastatin 20 mg plus ezetimibe 10 mg daily safely reduced the incidence of major atherosclerotic events.[85]

Non-steroidal Mineralocorticoid Receptor Antagonist

Mineralocorticoid receptor activation has been associated with pathologic effects in kidney disease and has been implicated in multiple inflammatory and fibrotic pathways.[86,87] The newer class of non-steroidal (NS) mineralocorticoid receptor antagonists (MRAs) are selective to the mineralocorticoid receptor, and pose a low risk of hyperkalemia even at lower eGFRs and have been shown to reduce albuminuria in DN.[88] The Finerenone in Reducing Kidney Failure and Disease Progression in Diabetic Kidney Disease (Fidelio-CKD) trial demonstrated that the novel NS MRA, Finerenone, reduced the risk for DKD progression and cardiovascular events as compared to placebo in patients with DKD. Guidelines recommend using NS MRAs as add-on therapy in patients with normal potassium levels < 4.8 who are already taking SGLT2is and RAASis, and who are at high risk from DKD progression as evidenced by albuminuria (>30 mcg/mg).[35]

SUMMARY

DKD, an all-encompassing term increasingly used to describe types of kidney failure that affect patients with diabetes, is a particularly formidable complication of diabetes and affects up to 40% of individuals with diabetes. With a better understanding of the pathophysiological mechanisms underlying DKD and with recent clinical trials showing promising therapeutic intervention, never before have we stood at the precipice of a meaningful impact on this public health threat. Challenges remain, however, with the implementation of, and sustained adherence to, these interventions on a population level.

CLINICS CARE POINTS

- DKD is asymptomatic in early stages and routine screening is important for early diagnosis.
- Diabetic patients should be screened annually for kidney disease by checking eGFRa nd UACR
- Lifestyle modification, good control of blood pressure and blood sugar remains cornerstone of DKD management.
- All DKD patients should be treated with an angiotensin-converting enzyme inhibitor or angiotensin II receptor blocker as tolerated.
- Type 2 diabetes and DKD pateints should be evaluated for treatment with SGLT-2 inhibitor, regardless of degee of glycemic control.
- Glucagon-like peptide-1 receptor agonists and non-steroidal mineralocorticoid receptor antagonists should be considered for add-on therapy.

FINANCIAL SUPPORT AND SPONSORSHIP

None.

CONFLICTS OF INTEREST

None.

ACKNOWLEDGMENTS

None.

REFERENCES

1. Federation ID. nternational Diabetes Federation. IDF Diabetes Atlas. 10th edn. Brussels, Belgium.
2. Centers for Disease Control and Prevention. National Diabetes Statistics Report 2022.
3. Lin E, Erickson KF. Payer Mix Among Patients Receiving Dialysis. JAMA 2020; 324(9):900–1.
4. Zimmet PZ. Diabetes and its drivers: the largest epidemic in human history? Clinical diabetes and endocrinology 2017;3(1):1–8.
5. Hill-Briggs F, Adler NE, Berkowitz SA, et al. Social determinants of health and diabetes: a scientific review. Diabetes Care 2021;44(1):258–79.
6. Koye DN, Magliano DJ, Nelson RG, et al. The global epidemiology of diabetes and kidney disease. Adv Chron Kidney Dis 2018;25(2):121–32.
7. Piccoli GB, Grassi G, Cabiddu G, et al. Diabetic kidney disease: a syndrome rather than a single disease. Rev Diabet Stud: Reg Dev Stud 2015;12(1–2):87.
8. Umanth K, Lewis J. Update on diabetic nephropathy: core curriculum. Am J Kidney Dis 2018;71(6):884–95.

9. Deshpande AD, Harris-Hayes M, Schootman M. Epidemiology of diabetes and diabetes-related complications. Phys Ther 2008;88(11):1254–64.

10. Thomas MC, Cooper ME, Zimmet P. Changing epidemiology of type 2 diabetes mellitus and associated chronic kidney disease. Nat Rev Nephrol 2016;12(2): 73–81.

11. Golestaneh L, Alvarez PJ, Reaven NL, et al. All-cause costs increase exponentially with increased chronic kidney disease stage. Am J Manag Care 2017; 23(10 Suppl):S163–72.

12. Folkerts K, Petruski-Ivleva N, Kelly A, et al. Annual health care resource utilization and cost among type 2 diabetes patients with newly recognized chronic kidney disease within a large US administrative claims database. J Manag Care Spec Pharm 2020;26(12):1506–16.

13. Perkins BA, Bebu I, de Boer IH, et al. Optimal Frequency of Urinary Albumin Screening in Type 1 Diabetes. Diabetes Care 2022;45(12):2943–9.

14. 11. Microvascular Complications and Foot Care: Standards of Medical Care in Diabetes-2019. Diabetes Care 2019;42(Suppl 1):S124–38. https://doi.org/10. 2337/dc19-S011 [published Online First: Epub Date]|.

15. Alicic RZ, Rooney MT, Tuttle KR. Diabetic kidney disease: challenges, progress, and possibilities. Clin J Am Soc Nephrol 2017;12(12):2032–45.

16. Pavkov ME, Knowler WC, Hanson RL, et al. Diabetic nephropathy in American Indians, with a special emphasis on the Pima Indians. Curr Diabetes Rep 2008; 8(6):486–93.

17. Jolly SE, Li S, Chen S-C, et al. Risk factors for chronic kidney disease among american indians and alaska natives–findings from the kidney early evaluation program. Am J Nephrol 2009;29(5):440–6.

18. Beckman JA, Creager MA. Vascular complications of diabetes. Circ Res 2016; 118(11):1771–85.

19. Wahba IM, Mak RH. Obesity and obesity-initiated metabolic syndrome: mechanistic links to chronic kidney disease. Clin J Am Soc Nephrol 2007;2(3):550–62.

20. Dronavalli S, Duka I, Bakris GL. The pathogenesis of diabetic nephropathy. Nat Clin Pract Endocrinol Metabol 2008;4(8):444–52.

21. Cao Z, Cooper ME. Pathogenesis of diabetic nephropathy. J Diabetes Investig 2011;2(4):243–7 [published Online First: Epub Date]|.

22. Lee K, He JC. AKI-to-CKD transition is a potential mechanism for non-albuminuric diabetic kidney disease. Faculty Reviews 2022;11. https://doi.org/10.12703/r/ 11-21.

23. Doshi SM, Friedman AN. Diagnosis and management of type 2 diabetic kidney disease. Clin J Am Soc Nephrol 2017;12(8):1366–73.

24. Furuichi K, Yuzawa Y, Shimizu M, et al. Nationwide multicentre kidney biopsy study of Japanese patients with type 2 diabetes. Nephrol Dial Transplant 2018; 33(1):138–48.

25. Lin JS, Susztak K. Podocytes: the Weakest Link in Diabetic Kidney Disease? Curr Diab Rep 2016;16(5):45 [published Online First: Epub Date]|.

26. Qazi M, Sawaf H, Ismail J, et al. Pathophysiology of Diabetic Kidney Disease. Nephrology 2022;102–13.

27. Meyer T, Bennett P, Nelson R. Podocyte number predicts long-term urinary albumin excretion in Pima Indians with type II diabetes and microalbuminuria. Diabetologia 1999;42(11):1341–4.

28. Nishad R, Tahaseen V, Kavvuri R, et al. Advanced-glycation end-products induce podocyte injury and contribute to proteinuria. Front Med 2021;8:685447.

29. Lentini P., Zanoli L., Ronco C., et al., The vascular disease of diabetic kidney disease, *Cardiorenal Medicine*, 2022. Online ahead of print.

30. Barton M, Tharaux P-L. Endothelin and the podocyte. Clin Kidney J 2012;5(1): 17–27.

31. Gurley SB, Coffman TM. The renin-angiotensin system and diabetic nephropathy. Semin Nephrol 2007;27(2):144–52. Elsevier.

32. Anders H-J, Huber TB, Isermann B, et al. CKD in diabetes: diabetic kidney disease versus nondiabetic kidney disease. Nat Rev Nephrol 2018;14(6):361–77.

33. Levin A, Stevens PE, Bilous RW, et al. Kidney Disease: Improving Global Outcomes (KDIGO) CKD Work Group. KDIGO 2012 clinical practice guideline for the evaluation and management of chronic kidney disease. Kidney Int Suppl 2013;3(1):1–150.

34. Penno G, Solini A, Orsi E, et al. Non-albuminuric renal impairment is a strong predictor of mortality in individuals with type 2 diabetes: the Renal Insufficiency And Cardiovascular Events (RIACE) Italian multicentre study. Diabetologia 2018; 61(11):2277–89.

35. de Boer IH, Khunti K, Sadusky T, et al. Diabetes management in chronic kidney disease: a consensus report by the American Diabetes Association (ADA) and Kidney Disease: Improving Global Outcomes (KDIGO). Kidney Int 2022;102(5): 974–89.

36. Rossing P, Caramori ML, Chan JC, et al. KDIGO 2022 Clinical Practice Guideline for Diabetes Management in Chronic Kidney Disease. Kidney Int 2022;102(5): S1–127.

37. Delgado C, Baweja M, Crews DC, et al. A Unifying Approach for GFR Estimation: Recommendations of the NKF-ASN Task Force on Reassessing the Inclusion of Race in Diagnosing Kidney Disease. Am J Kidney Dis 2022;79(2):268–88 [published Online First: Epub Date]].

38. Pichaiwong W, Hudkins KL, Wietecha T, et al. Reversibility of structural and functional damage in a model of advanced diabetic nephropathy. J Am Soc Nephrol 2013;24(7):1088–102.

39. Wang J, Xiang H, Lu Y, et al. New progress in drugs treatment of diabetic kidney disease. Biomed Pharmacother 2021;141:111918.

40. Rikin S, Deccy S, Zhang C, et al. Care Gaps in Sodium-Glucose Cotransporter-2 Inhibitor and Renin Angiotensin System Inhibitor Prescriptions for Patients with Diabetic Kidney Disease. J Gen Intern Med 2022;1–7.

41. Friedman AN, Kaplan LM, le Roux CW, et al. Management of obesity in adults with CKD. J Am Soc Nephrol 2021;32(4):777–90.

42. Wapstra FH, Van Goor H, Navis G, et al. Antiproteinuric effect predicts renal protection by angiotensin-converting enzyme inhibition in rats with established adriamycin nephrosis. Clinical science 1996;90(5):393–401.

43. Vogt L, Waanders F, Boomsma F, et al. Effects of dietary sodium and hydrochlorothiazide on the antiproteinuric efficacy of losartan. J Am Soc Nephrol 2008; 19(5):999–1007.

44. de Boer IH, Khunti K, Sadusky T, et al. Diabetes management in chronic kidney disease: a consensus report by the American Diabetes Association (ADA) and Kidney Disease: Improving Global Outcomes (KDIGO). Diabetes Care 2022; 45(12):3075–90.

45. Cheung AK, Chang TI, Cushman WC, et al. KDIGO 2021 clinical practice guideline for the management of blood pressure in chronic kidney disease. Kidney Int 2021;99(3):S1–87.

46. Association AH. Guideline on the primary prevention of cardiovascular disease. Circulation 2019;140:e596–646.

47. Levey AS, Greene T, Beck GJ, et al. Dietary protein restriction and the progression of chronic renal disease: what have all of the results of the MDRD study shown? J Am Soc Nephrol 1999;10(11):2426–39.

48. Kasiske BL, Lakatua J, Ma JZ, et al. A meta-analysis of the effects of dietary protein restriction on the rate of decline in renal function. Am J Kidney Dis 1998; 31(6):954–61.

49. Pedrini MT, Levey AS, Lau J, et al. The effect of dietary protein restriction on the progression of diabetic and nondiabetic renal diseases: a meta-analysis. Annals of internal medicine 1996;124(7):627–32.

50. Ikizler TA, Cuppari L. The 2020 updated KDOQI clinical practice guidelines for nutrition in chronic kidney disease. Blood Purif 2021;50(4–5):667–71.

51. Care D. Care in Diabetesd2019. Diabetes Care 2019;42(1):S13–28.

52. Bundy JD, Li C, Stuchlik P, et al. Systolic blood pressure reduction and risk of cardiovascular disease and mortality: a systematic review and network meta-analysis. JAMA cardiology 2017;2(7):775–81.

53. Wright JT Jr, Bakris G, Greene T, et al. Effect of blood pressure lowering and antihypertensive drug class on progression of hypertensive kidney disease: results from the AASK trial. JAMA 2002;288(19):2421–31 [published Online First: Epub Date]|.

54. Intensive blood-glucose control with sulphonylureas or insulin compared with conventional treatment and risk of complications in patients with type 2 diabetes (UKPDS 33). UK Prospective Diabetes Study (UKPDS) Group. Lancet 1998; 352(9131):837–53.

55. Group AS. Effects of intensive blood-pressure control in type 2 diabetes mellitus. N Engl J Med 2010;362(17):1575–85.

56. Group AC. Intensive blood glucose control and vascular outcomes in patients with type 2 diabetes. N Engl J Med 2008;358(24):2560–72.

57. Duckworth W, Abraira C, Moritz T, et al. Glucose control and vascular complications in veterans with type 2 diabetes. N Engl J Med 2009;360(2):129–39.

58. Nathan D. for the Diabetes Control and Complications Trial/Epidemiology of Diabetes Interventions and Complications (DCCT/EDIC) study research group. Intensive diabetes treatment and cardiovascular disease in patients with type 1 diabetes. N Engl J Med 2005;353:2643–53.

59. Holman RR, Paul SK, Bethel MA, et al. 10-year follow-up of intensive glucose control in type 2 diabetes. N Engl J Med 2008;359(15):1577–89.

60. Nathan D, Genuth S, Lachin J, et al. The effect of intensive treatment of diabetes on the development and progression of long-term complications in insulin-dependent diabetes mellitus. N Engl J Med 1993;329(14):977–86.

61. Lee AK, Warren B, Lee CJ, et al. The association of severe hypoglycemia with incident cardiovascular events and mortality in adults with type 2 diabetes. Diabetes Care 2018;41(1):104–11.

62. Group UPDS. Intensive blood-glucose control with sulphonylureas or insulin compared with conventional treatment and risk of complications in patients with type 2 diabetes (UKPDS 33). Lancet 1998;352(9131):837–53.

63. Lazarus B, Wu A, Shin J-I, et al. Association of metformin use with risk of lactic acidosis across the range of kidney function: a community-based cohort study. JAMA Intern Med 2018;178(7):903–10.

64. Scheen A.J., Cardiovascular and renal protection with sodium-glucose co-transporter type 2 inhibitors: new paradigm in type 2 diabetes management and potentially beyond, *Ann Transl Med*, 7 (Suppl 3), 2019, S132.

65. Bays H. Sodium Glucose Co-transporter Type 2 (SGLT2) Inhibitors: Targeting the Kidney to Improve Glycemic Control in Diabetes Mellitus. Diabetes Ther 2013; 4(2):195–220 [published Online First: Epub Date]|.

66. Vallon V, Verma S. Effects of SGLT2 Inhibitors on Kidney and Cardiovascular Function. Annu Rev Physiol 2021;83:503–28 [published Online First: Epub Date]|.

67. van Bommel EJ, Muskiet MH, Tonneijck L, et al. SGLT2 Inhibition in the Diabetic Kidney-From Mechanisms to Clinical Outcome. Clin J Am Soc Nephrol 2017; 12(4):700–10 [published Online First: Epub Date]|.

68. Rabizadeh S, Nakhjavani M, Esteghamati A. Cardiovascular and Renal Benefits of SGLT2 Inhibitors: A Narrative Review. Int J Endocrinol Metab 2019;17(2): e84353 [published Online First: Epub Date]|.

69. Kidokoro K, Cherney DZI, Bozovic A, et al. Evaluation of Glomerular Hemodynamic Function by Empagliflozin in Diabetic Mice Using In Vivo Imaging. Circulation 2019;140(4):303–15 [published Online First: Epub Date]|.

70. Patel AB, Mistry K, Verma A. DAPA-CKD: Significant Victory for CKD with or without Diabetes. Trends Endocrinol Metab 2021;32(6):335–7 [published Online First: Epub Date]|.

71. Yau K, Dharia A, Alrowiyti I, et al. Prescribing SGLT2 Inhibitors in Patients With CKD: Expanding Indications and Practical Considerations. Kidney Int Rep 2022;7(7):1463–76 [published Online First: Epub Date]|.

72. Toyama T, Neuen BL, Jun M, et al. Effect of SGLT2 inhibitors on cardiovascular, renal and safety outcomes in patients with type 2 diabetes mellitus and chronic kidney disease: A systematic review and meta-analysis. Diabetes Obes Metab 2019;21(5):1237–50 [published Online First: Epub Date]|.

73. Shaman AM, Bain SC, Bakris GL, et al. Effect of the Glucagon-Like Peptide-1 Receptor Agonists Semaglutide and Liraglutide on Kidney Outcomes in Patients With Type 2 Diabetes: Pooled Analysis of SUSTAIN 6 and LEADER. Circulation 2022;145(8):575–85.

74. Górriz JL, Soler MJ, Navarro-González JF, et al. GLP-1 receptor agonists and diabetic kidney disease: a call of attention to nephrologists. J Clin Med 2020; 9(4):947.

75. Nauck MA, Stewart MW, Perkins C, et al. Efficacy and safety of once-weekly GLP-1 receptor agonist albiglutide (HARMONY 2): 52 week primary endpoint results from a randomised, placebo-controlled trial in patients with type 2 diabetes mellitus inadequately controlled with diet and exercise. Diabetologia 2016;59(2): 266–74 [published Online First: Epub Date]|.

76. Verma S, Bhatt DL, Bain SC, et al. Effect of liraglutide on cardiovascular events in patients with type 2 diabetes mellitus and polyvascular disease: results of the LEADER trial. Circulation 2018;137(20):2179–83.

77. Gerstein HC, Colhoun HM, Dagenais GR, et al. Dulaglutide and cardiovascular outcomes in type 2 diabetes (REWIND): a double-blind, randomised placebo-controlled trial. Lancet 2019;394(10193):121–30.

78. Parving H-H, Lehnert H, Bröchner-Mortensen J, et al. The effect of irbesartan on the development of diabetic nephropathy in patients with type 2 diabetes. N Engl J Med 2001;345(12):870–8.

79. Lewis E, Hunsicker LG, Bain RP, Rohde RD, Collaborative Study Group. The effect of angiotensin-converting enzyme inhibition on diabetic nephropathy. N Engl J Med 1993;329:1456–62.

80. Ravera M, Ratto E, Vettoretti S, et al. Prevention and treatment of diabetic ne-phropathy: the program for irbesartan mortality and morbidity evaluation. J Am Soc Nephrol 2005;16(3 suppl 1):S48–52.

81. Brenner BM, Cooper ME, De Zeeuw D, et al. Effects of losartan on renal and car-diovascular outcomes in patients with type 2 diabetes and nephropathy. N Engl J Med 2001;345(12):861–9.

82. Björck S, Mulec H, Johnsen SA, et al. Renal protective effect of enalapril in dia-betic nephropathy. Br Med J 1992;304(6823):339–43.

83. Grassi G. The ROADMAP trial: olmesartan for the delay or prevention of microal-buminuria in type 2 diabetes. Expert Opin Pharmacother 2011;12(15):2421–4 [published Online First: Epub Date]|.

84. Betteridge J. Benefits of lipid-lowering therapy in patients with type 2 diabetes mellitus. Am J Med 2005;118(Suppl 12A):10–5 [published Online First: Epub Date]|.

85. Baigent C, Landray MJ, Reith C, et al. The effects of lowering LDL cholesterol with simvastatin plus ezetimibe in patients with chronic kidney disease (Study of Heart and Renal Protection): a randomised placebo-controlled trial. Lancet 2011; 377(9784):2181–92 [published Online First: Epub Date]|.

86. Luther JM, Fogo AB. The role of mineralocorticoid receptor activation in kidney inflammation and fibrosis. Kidney Int Suppl (2011) 2022;12(1):63–8 [published Online First: Epub Date]|.

87. Nakamura T, Girerd S, Jaisser F, et al. Nonepithelial mineralocorticoid receptor activation as a determinant of kidney disease. Kidney Int Suppl (2011) 2022; 12(1):12–8 [published Online First: Epub Date]|.

88. Epstein M, Kovesdy CP, Clase CM, et al. Aldosterone, Mineralocorticoid Receptor Activation, and CKD: A Review of Evolving Treatment Paradigms. Am J Kidney Dis 2022;80(5):658–66 [published Online First: Epub Date]|.

Overview of Renal Transplantation for Primary Care Physicians
Workup, Complications, and Management

Priyanka Jethwani, MBBS[a,b]

KEYWORDS

- Kidney • Transplant • Immunosuppression • Donation • Primary care

KEY POINTS

- Kidney transplantation is the treatment of choice for end-stage kidney disease with an increasing pool of kidney transplant recipients.
- There is a role for the primary care physicians in the workup and long-term management of kidney transplant recipients.
- Transplant recipients need lifelong immunosuppressing medications that put them at risk of side effects, drug-drug interactions, and infections.
- Cardiovascular disease and malignancy are the foremost causes of death in these patients, and there is need for aggressive modification of risk factors and screening.

INTRODUCTION

The last several decades have seen a rising burden of kidney disease in the United States, with as many as 807,920 individuals with end-stage kidney disease (ESKD) in 2020.[1] Kidney transplantation offers patients improved quality as well as longevity of life and so remains the treatment of choice for ESKD in eligible candidates. There is an increasing number of solid organ transplants in the United States every year with 25,499 kidney transplants performed last year alone based on Organ Procurement & Transplantation Network national data as of December 31, 2022.

With the success of endeavors to prolong allograft and patient survival, the transplant recipient pool continues to expand. As a result, the long-term care of transplant recipients is no longer restricted to transplant centers, with most centers referring patients out to general nephrologists and primary care physicians as early as 6 months after transplant. This calls for increased involvement and comfort among primary care

[a] James D Eason Transplant Institute, Methodist University Hospital, 1265 Union Avenue, Memphis, TN 38104, USA; [b] Department of Surgery, University of Tennessee Health Sciences Center, 1211 Union Avenue, Memphis, TN 38104, USA
E-mail address: priyanka.jethwani@mlh.org

Med Clin N Am 107 (2023) 707–716
https://doi.org/10.1016/j.mcna.2023.03.008
0025-7125/23/© 2023 Elsevier Inc. All rights reserved.

physicians (PCPs) with long-term management of these patients with a refined understanding of various aspects of their care.

KIDNEY TRANSPLANT WORKUP FOR THE PRIMARY CARE PHYSICIAN
Evaluation of Candidates for Transplant

Kidney transplantation is indicated for patients with advanced, irreversible kidney disease. Patients are referred to the transplant center, usually by their general nephrologist, for pre-kidney-transplant evaluation at an estimated glomerular filtration rate (eGFR) of around 25 mL/min/1.72 m^2. This proactive approach allows for sufficient time to complete pretransplant testing and timely listing. Since the change in organ allocation system in 2014, patients can actively be listed for a kidney transplant once their eGFR falls below 20 mL/min and start to gain wait-time on the kidney transplant list even prior to starting dialysis. For patients already on dialysis, wait-time accrues since the start of dialysis. In general, it is best to avoid referring patients with higher eGFR to the transplant center so as not to burden already taxed resources.

The overall purpose of the initial kidney transplant evaluation is to

- Determine whether the patient will benefit from a kidney transplant; is it likely to improve quality of life and increase survival?
- Review medical history in detail to determine risk factors that need to be modified and pre-existing conditions that need to be monitored if the patient were to receive a transplant.
- Educate the patient and accompanying family members or friends about the kidney transplant process and present an opportunity to ask clarifying questions.
- Encourage the patient to investigate the possibility of finding a living kidney donor.

Once the initial evaluation visit is complete, patients undergo extensive testing depending on age, comorbid conditions, and center-specific requirements. Some testing is mandated to be done through the transplant center itself, but some tests may be coordinated by the transplant center through the PCPs office. Results of age-appropriate cancer screening tests are an essential part of a complete evaluation, and the primary care office can play a vital role in ensuring that patients are up to date with age-appropriate cancer screening and that results are shared with the transplant center, ideally along with the patient referral.

Primary care physicians enjoy a special rapport with patients and families and can play a unique role in advocating early on for living kidney donation to accompanying friends and family members. This not only minimizes time spent on the waiting list but also helps reduce burden on the already limited cadaveric organ pool. Once the potential recipient has begun evaluation at a center, willing donors can come forward and be evaluated for suitability to donate. With the option for kidney paired donation via national and institution-based registries, donors are no longer restricted by tissue compatibility. Therefore, no willing donor should be excluded as an option based on blood type. Short- and long-term survival of both living related and living unrelated kidney transplants are superior to those of cadaveric kidneys. Many resources are available online to share with patients and potential donors more information regarding living donation to get an early start on finding a living donor, such as https://unos.org/transplant/living-donation/.

Another area of opportunity for the PCP in the pre-kidney-transplant workup is ensuring that patients are fully immunized based on United States Preventive Services Task Force (USPSTF) guidelines for the general population prior to the transplant.

Because of induction immunosuppression at the time of transplant as well as life-long maintenance immunosuppression, vaccine effectiveness may be variable after transplantation. Policies regarding COVID-19 vaccination vary across the nation, and even if not mandated, it is certainly recommended that patients receive the full vaccination series before transplant. Smoking cessation should also be discussed and encouraged, and PCPs can prepare patients with resources and tools to facilitate smoking cessation.

COMMON POST-TRANSPLANT COMPLICATIONS
Acute Kidney Injury

Evaluation of acute kidney injury (AKI) in a transplant recipient can be challenging. The differential diagnosis is broad, and although allograft rejection is always on the list, it may not always be the top contender. The most common causes of AKI more than 6 months out from kidney transplantation in no specific order include volume depletion, hemodynamic insult, urinary tract infection, BK virus nephropathy, transplant renal artery stenosis, acute rejection, chronic rejection, recurrence of primary kidney disease, and drug-induced injury especially in the setting of calcineurin inhibitor (CNI; discussed in detail below).

In general, the approach to AKI in the transplant recipient involves detailed history-taking with focus on ascertaining medication adherence, blood work including comprehensive metabolic panel, urinalysis with microscopic evaluation, urine protein-creatinine ratio, immunosuppressive drug levels, and renal allograft ultrasound (US) with Dopplers. In the absence of obvious causes of AKI that fail to resolve with hydration, adjustment of drug levels, and treatment of any underlying infection, or in cases of new proteinuria accompanied by rising creatinine, patients should be directed back to the transplant center for urgent evaluation and kidney biopsy.

Immunosuppressive Medications and Drug-Drug Interactions

Transplant recipients require immunosuppressive medications for the life of their allograft, making it essential for primary care physicians to be aware of their side effects and potential for drug-drug interactions. While each patient has slightly different immunosuppressive needs, most transplant centers use CNIs (cyclosporine or tacrolimus) as the mainstay therapy in addition to an antimetabolite agent (azathioprine or mycophenolate mofetil) with or without low-dose prednisone. In certain cases, mammalian target of rapamycin inhibitors (mTORIs) such as sirolimus or everolimus may be used to minimize exposure to CNIs due to their nephrotoxic side effects. Additionally, an intravenous agent, belatacept, is now being used more and more in various combinations with other agents for maintenance immunosuppression due to better long-term graft outcomes.[2] **Table 1** shows a review of mechanisms of action and side effects of commonly used immunosuppressants. **Table 2** shows a review of common drug-drug interactions to monitor for with ongoing CNI therapy due to metabolism via the hepatic and gastrointestinal CYP3A enzyme system. Care must be exercised when starting or stopping any of the listed medications as they may result in drug toxicity or subtherapeutic levels that can cause rejection.

Common Infections and Prophylaxis

Owing to the need for chronic immunosuppression, transplant recipients are at increased lifetime risk of infections. The risk is highest within the first 3 to 6 months after surgery and decreases with time.

Within 30 days of transplant, health care–associated infections are the most common ones such as surgical site infections, urinary tract infections, central line–

Table 1
Commonly used immunosuppressive agents and their mechanism of action and side effects

Immunosuppressive Agent	Mechanism of Action	Side Effects

Calcineurin Inhibitors
  Tacrolimus (Prograf,
    Astagraf, Envarsus-XR)
  Cyclosporine (Neoral,
    Sandimmune)
	Binds FK506 binding protein
	  to inhibit signal one
	Binds cyclophilin to inhibit
	  signal one
		Hyperkalemia, hypertension,
		  nephrotoxicity,
		  neurotoxicity (eg,
		  headaches, tremors,
		  neuropathy, seizures),
		  diabetes, alopecia
		Dyslipidemia, gingival
		  hyperplasia, hirsutism,
		  gout

Purine Antimetabolites
  Azathioprine
  Mycophenolate mofetil
    (Cellcept)
  Mycophenolic acid
    (Myfortic)
	Purine analog
	Inosine monophosphate
	  dehydrogenase (IMPDH)
	  inhibitor
		Cholestatic hepatitis,
		  myelosuppression
		  especially in combination
		  with allopurinol
		Bone marrow suppression,
		  gastrointestinal issues (eg,
		  abdominal pain, diarrhea,
		  gastritis, nausea)

mTORIs
  Sirolimus
  Everolimus
	Binds FK506 binding protein
	  to inhibit target of
	  rapamycin (TOR) and
	  inhibits signal three
		Dyslipidemia, hepatic artery
		  thrombosis,
		  myelosuppression, poor
		  wound healing, pulmonary
		  fibrosis, rash, ulcerations,
		  edema, proteinuria

Belatacept (Nulojix, IV)	Selective costimulation
	  blocker, binds CD80 and
	  CD86 on APCs blocking
	  signal two
		Black box warning against
		  use in EBV naive patients
		  due to risk of PTLD
		PTLD in EBV naive patients
		Increased risk of cell-
		  mediated rejection

Abbreviations: APCs, antigen presenting cells; EBV, Epstein-Barr virus; PTLD, posttransplant lymphoproliferative disorder.

associated blood-stream infections, donor-derived infection, and clostridium difficile infection. Between 30 days and 1 year, most infections are opportunistic in the setting of overimmunosuppression. Beyond 1 year, patients are most likely to develop community-acquired infections, and late development of opportunistic infections should prompt workup for underlying malignancy or other secondarily immunosuppressing states.

Owing to the high risk of either reactivation of latent cytomegalovirus (CMV) infection or new primary CMV infection from the donor organ, patients are given prophylactic therapy with valganciclovir for 3 months or 6 months, respectively. While uncommonly seen in the general population, CMV infection has a spectrum of manifestations ranging from viremia to gastrointestinal, bone marrow, or pulmonary tissue invasive disease.

Patients also receive 6 months to 1 year of prophylaxis against *Pneumocystis jirovecii* infection, which can cause severe pneumonia in immunocompromised individuals. The prophylactic antibiotic of choice is trimethoprim/sulfamethoxazole, but alternative agents such as dapsone, atovaquone, or inhaled pentamidine may be used in the setting of drug intolerance or sulfa allergy.

Table 2
Drug interactions to monitor with CNIs

Inhibitors of Cytochrome P450 (Increase CNI Levels)	Inducers of Cytochrome P450 (Decrease CNI Levels)
Antiarrhythmics	Antiepileptic Drugs
Amiodarone, dronedarone	Barbiturates, phenytoin, fosphenytoin,
Antibiotics	carbamazepine, valproic acid
Macrolides (clarithromycin, erythromycin)	Rifampin, rifabutin, rifapentine
Antifungals (azoles)	St John's Wort
Fluconazole, itraconazole, voriconazole	Efavirenz, nevirapine, Etravirine
Clotrimazole, ketoconazole	Bosentan
Calcium channel blockers	Modafinil
Verapamil, diltiazem	Nafcillin
Protease Inhibitors	Cholestyramine
Ritonavir, darunavir, atazanavir	
Others	
Grapefruit, grapefruit juice	
Isoniazid	
Cimetidine	
Cobicistat	
Conivaptan	

This is not an exhaustive list.

Urinary tract infections most commonly occur in kidney transplant recipients within 6 months after transplant.[3] This is due to the lack of a natural antireflux valve between the transplanted ureter and bladder allowing reflux of urine and relatively shorter length of ureter that facilitates ascending infection. Cystitis is usually treated with oral antibiotics, but acute pyelonephritis can be allograft- and life-threatening and is recommended to be treated inpatient with parenteral antibiotics.

No consensus statement or guidelines exist regarding screening for and treating asymptomatic bacteriuria after the first few weeks of transplant. Several studies report no benefit to treating asymptomatic bacteriuria and document emergence of antibiotic resistance due to this practice.[4,5]

A more detailed discussion about common and uncommon infections affecting the transplant population is out of the scope of this publication but is beautifully reviewed in a recent article.[6]

CHRONIC MEDICAL CONDITIONS AND MANAGEMENT
Cardiovascular Disease

While kidney transplantation provides cardiovascular mortality benefit compared to remaining on long-term dialysis, it represents a state of accelerated atherogenic risk. It remains the leading cause of death in up to 50% to 60% of transplant recipients,[7] with cardiovascular disease appearing up to 20 years earlier in kidney transplant recipients than that in the general population.[8]

The spectrum of cardiac disease after transplantation ranges across coronary artery disease, heart failure, cardiac arrhythmias, and pulmonary hypertension. Owing to a prior history of chronic kidney disease and years on dialysis, patients suffer from both traditional cardiac risk factors as well as posttransplantation nontraditional risk factors that compound overall cardiac risk.[9] Traditional risk factors include hypertension, diabetes, smoking, and hyperlipidemia. However, transplant recipients are also exposed to immunosuppressive agents such as CNIs and mTORIs that are both atherogenic and diabetogenic. Other nontraditional risk factors include increased oxidative stress[10] and inflammation as well as mineral bone disease,[11] which contribute to the cardiovascular risk. In addition, anywhere between 10% and 60% of kidney transplant recipients report obesity[12] with as much as 15 kg of weight gain within the first year after transplant,[13,14] which again contributes to overall risk.

Unfortunately, there are no cardiovascular risk calculators to estimate individualized risk for transplant recipients, and there lacks a body of evidence or specialized guidelines regarding prevention and treatment of cardiovascular disease in these patients. As such, it is recommended to have a proactive approach toward aggressive modification of cardiovascular risk factors as is done in the general population. Patients should be counseled for smoking cessation as well as diet and exercise. Statin therapy is recommended for all solid organ transplant recipients. The Assessment of Lescol in Renal Transplantation(ALeRT) trial demonstrated a reduction in cardiac death and nonfatal myocardial infarctions with fluvastatin in kidney transplant recipients.[15] Other statins can be used interchangeably starting at the lowest dose to avoid interactions with CNIs with subsequent maximization.

Hypertension

Hypertension in kidney transplant recipients is common and often multifactorial because of pretransplant hypertension, as a side effect of CNIs and chronic steroid use and due to progressive allograft dysfunction. Hillebrand and colleagues demonstrated improved allograft survival in patients with controlled versus uncontrolled blood pressure (BP; 106 ± 2.4 months vs 100 ± 2.2 months, $P < .05$), with control defined as BP < 130/80 mm Hg.[16] In another study, adjusted for other variables, each 10-mm Hg systolic BP increase was shown to be associated with an increased relative risk of graft failure (relative risk 1.12, $P < .0001$).[17] While no large clinical trials exist to determine ideal BP goals in this cohort of patients, the KDIGO clinical practice guidelines of 2021 recommend a BP goal of <130/80 mm Hg for kidney transplant recipients. Dihydropyridine calcium channel blockers and angiotensin-converting enzyme inhibitors/angiotensin receptor blockers (ACEI/ARBs) are recommended as first-line agents.

Posttransplant Diabetes Mellitus

Kidney transplant recipients are at risk of developing posttransplant diabetes mellitus (PTDM), with cumulative incidence reported up to 29% at 5 years after transplant in a multicenter study.[18] Individuals who develop PTDM are at higher risk of death-censored graft failure and death than recipients that do not.[19] In addition, there is an estimated $21,500 extra cost to Medicare per newly diabetic patient by 2 years after transplant.[20]

The following modifiable risk factors for the development of PTDM have been identified: higher body mass index, weight gain after transplant, hepatitis C virus infection, immunosuppressive medications, hypomagnesemia, decreased physical activity, and unhealthy diet. Patients should, therefore, be counseled about aggressive lifestyle modification with diet and exercise to combat some of these risk factors. CNIs, especially tacrolimus, increase the risk of PTDM by way of direct pancreatic beta cell toxicity, an effect which is less pronounced with cyclosporine. Patients on tacrolimus may be directed back to the transplant center to consider transition to either cyclosporine or any alternative medication to minimize this effect. Posttransplant weight gain should be managed aggressively with consideration of medical weight loss with glucagon-like peptide-1 (GLP-1) agonists or referral for evaluation regarding bariatric surgery in discussion with the transplant center.

Treatment of diabetes in the transplant recipient is similar to that in the general population. In addition, there is emerging data regarding sodium-glucose cotransporter 2 inhibitor (SGLT2i) use in the transplant population with evidence that SGLT2i use has a lower risk of primary composite outcome of all-cause mortality, death-censored graft loss, or serum creatinine doubling in kidney transplant recipients than in the control group in the multivariate and propensity score–matched models (adjusted hazard ratio, 0.43 (0.24–0.78); $P = .006$, adjusted hazard ratio, 0.45 (0.24–0.85); $P = .013$, respectively).[21] SGLT2i should be initiated with careful monitoring of kidney function, hydration, and keeping in mind individual risk of urinary tract infections.

Malignancy in Transplant Recipients

Cancer is the second most common cause of mortality after cardiovascular diseases in solid organ transplant recipients with a two- to four-fold increase in cancer risk compared to the general population.[22–24] This increase, however, is not uniform for all cancer types with some cancer incidence not being affected by kidney transplantation, for example, breast, prostate, ovarian, cervical, and brain cancers.[25–27]

The increased risk of de novo and recurrent cancer in transplant recipients is multifactorial and attributed to oncogenic viruses as well as altered T-cell immunity. In Western populations, nonmelanoma skin cancer is the most common type, comprising more than 50% of all post-kidney-transplant malignancies.[28–30] All kidney transplant recipients are advised to visit a dermatologist annually for complete skin examinations and wear sunscreen when exposed to the sun.

A number of viruses predispose transplant recipients to specific malignancies, including Epstein-Barr virus (EBV) (associated with lymphomas), human herpes virus 8 (lymphomas and Kaposi sarcoma), hepatitis viruses B and C (hepatocellular carcinoma), and human papillomaviruses (cervical, penile, and vulvar cancers). A 10-year observational study showed an 11.8-fold increase in the risk of developing posttransplant lymphoproliferative disorder (PTLD) in transplant recipients compared to the general population, with the highest incidence within the first year.[31] Risk was noted to be highest in EBV seronegative patients.[32]

In the absence of formal consensus guidelines for cancer screening in transplant patients, primary care physicians are urged to follow cancer screening guidelines for the general population as determined by USPSTF. Physicians should play close attention to symptoms of unprecedented weight loss, fevers, headaches, abdominal discomfort, and chills and obtain computed tomography imaging to look for lymphadenopathy that might be consistent with PTLD. Hematuria with or without erythrocytosis in a kidney transplant recipient should be evaluated with US imaging of both the native and transplanted kidney to rule out malignant transformation of renal cysts. If diagnosed with a malignancy, patients should be directed back to the transplant clinic for consideration of modification of immunosuppressive therapy.

Contraception, Family Planning, and Pregnancy

End-stage renal disease is associated with impaired fertility, but a majority of women regain their fertility within 1 year after transplantation. Women should be counseled at every opportunity before and after transplantation regarding the importance of a reliable method of contraception to prevent unwanted pregnancy. Owing to the teratogenic effects of mycophenolate mofetil, patients are counseled to maintain contraception while on it. Although all hormonal contraceptives are acceptable in patients with good allograft function and well-controlled BP, intrauterine devices or depot progesterone preparations are recommended because of the increased thrombotic risk and risk of hypertension with combined oral contraceptive pills.[33]

The decision to plan a pregnancy should be discussed with the transplant center and is generally only recommended at least 1 year after transplantation if posttransplant course has been relatively stable and rejection-free with SCr < 1.5 without significant proteinuria and well-controlled BPs.[34] Patients wishing to conceive should be switched from mycophenolate mofetil to azathioprine, which along with tacrolimus and prednisone is safe in pregnancy, for at least 3 months before discontinuing contraception.

Pregnancy should be monitored closely by high-risk obstetrics along with the transplant center, with a close eye on tacrolimus levels that fluctuate significantly with change in total circulating plasma volume and placental metabolism of the drug. Breastfeeding and vaginal delivery are not contraindicated in transplant recipients.

Immunization Guidelines

Ideally, all immunization should be completed before transplantation. After the transplant, recipients should wait at least 3 to 6 months before receiving most vaccines because of decreased efficacy of vaccination immediately after induction immunosuppression given at the time of surgery. The inactivated influenza vaccine can be administered as early as 1 month after transplant. Live attenuated vaccines in general should be avoided after transplantation.

Detailed recommendations regarding each individual vaccine can be reviewed in the most recent immunization update from the American Society of Transplantation Infectious Diseases Community of Practice.[35]

SUMMARY

The annually increasing volume of kidney transplants and improved mortality rates have led to a significant expansion of the total transplant recipient pool. Primary care physicians must take on a more active role in the long-term care of these patients for better management of chronic transplant-specific medical conditions.

CLINICS CARE POINTS

- Patients with kidney disease should be referred to the transplant center when their estimated glomerular filtration rate is at or around 25 mL/min/m².
- Living kidney donation should be discussed, and resource materials shared.
- Transplant recipients are at increased risk of cardiovascular disease due to hypertension, diabetes, obesity, and the atherogenic profile of immunosuppressive medications.
- Blood pressure target is <130/80 mm Hg, and statin use is recommended along with aggressive lifestyle modification.
- Malignancies are two- to four-fold more common in transplant recipients; most common malignancies are nonmelanoma skin cancers, renal cancer, and lymphoma.

DISCLOSURE

The authors have nothing to disclose.

REFERENCES

1. United States Renal Data System. 2022 USRDS annual data report: epidemiology of kidney disease in the United States. Bethesda, MD: National Institutes

of Health, National Institute of Diabetes and Digestive and Kidney Diseases; 2022.

2. Vincenti F, Rostaing L, Grinyo J, et al. Belatacept and Long-Term Outcomes in Kidney Transplantation. N Engl J Med 2016;374(4):333–43.

3. Veroux M, Giuffrida G, Corona D, et al. Infective complications in renal allograft recipients: epidemiology and outcome. Transplant Proc 2008;40(6):1873–6.

4. Origüen J, López-Medrano F, Fernández-Ruiz M, et al. Should Asymptomatic Bacteriuria Be Systematically Treated in Kidney Transplant Recipients? Results From a Randomized Controlled Trial. Am J Transplant 2016;16(10):2943–53.

5. Coussement J, Scemla A, Abramowicz D, et al. Antibiotics for asymptomatic bacteriuria in kidney transplant recipients. Cochrane Database Syst Rev 2018; 2(2):Cd011357.

6. Agrawal A, Ison MG, Danziger-Isakov L. Long-Term Infectious Complications of Kidney Transplantation. Clin J Am Soc Nephrol 2022;17(2):286–95.

7. Ojo AO. Cardiovascular Complications After Renal Transplantation and Their Prevention. Transplantation 2006;82(5):603–11.

8. Aakhus S, Dahl K, Widerøe TE. Cardiovascular morbidity and risk factors in renal transplant patients. Nephrol Dial Transplant 1999;14(3):648–54.

9. Birdwell K.A. and Park M., Post-transplant cardiovascular disease, *Clin J Am Soc Nephrol*, 16 (12), 2021, 1878-1889.

10. Ducloux D, Kazory A, Chalopin JM. Predicting coronary heart disease in renal transplant recipients: a prospective study. Kidney Int 2004;66(1):441–7.

11. Seifert ME, Hruska KA. The Kidney-Vascular-Bone Axis in the Chronic Kidney Disease-Mineral Bone Disorder. Transplantation 2016;100(3):497–505.

12. Lentine KL, Rocca-Rey LA, Bacchi G, et al. Obesity and cardiac risk after kidney transplantation: experience at one center and comprehensive literature review. Transplantation 2008;86(2):303–12.

13. Baum CL, Thielke K, Westin E, et al. Predictors of weight gain and cardiovascular risk in a cohort of racially diverse kidney transplant recipients. Nutrition 2002; 18(2):139–46.

14. Friedman AN, Miskulin DC, Rosenberg IH, et al. Demographics and trends in overweight and obesity in patients at time of kidney transplantation. Am J Kidney Dis 2003;41(2):480–7.

15. Holdaas H, Fellström B, Jardine AG, et al. Effect of fluvastatin on cardiac outcomes in renal transplant recipients: a multicentre, randomised, placebo-controlled trial. Lancet 2003;361(9374):2024–31.

16. Hillebrand U, Suwelack BM, Loley K, et al. Blood pressure, antihypertensive treatment, and graft survival in kidney transplant patients. Transpl Int 2009;22(11): 1073–80.

17. Kasiske BL, Anjum S, Shah R, et al. Hypertension after kidney transplantation. Am J Kidney Dis 2004;43(6):1071–81.

18. Malik RF, Jia Y, Mansour SG, et al. Post-transplant Diabetes Mellitus in Kidney Transplant Recipients: A Multicenter Study. Kidney360 2021;2(8):1296–307.

19. Kasiske BL, Snyder JJ, Gilbertson D, et al. Diabetes mellitus after kidney transplantation in the United States. Am J Transplant 2003;3(2):178–85.

20. Woodward RS, Schnitzler MA, Baty J, et al. Incidence and cost of new onset diabetes mellitus among U.S. wait-listed and transplanted renal allograft recipients. Am J Transplant 2003;3(5):590–8.

21. Lim JH, Kwon S, Jeon Y, et al. The Efficacy and Safety of SGLT2 Inhibitor in Diabetic Kidney Transplant Recipients. Transplantation 2022;106(9):e404–12.

22. Vajdic CM, McDonald SP, McCredie MR, et al. Cancer incidence before and after kidney transplantation. JAMA 2006;296(23):2823–31.
23. Villeneuve PJ, Schaubel DE, Fenton SS, et al. Cancer incidence among Canadian kidney transplant recipients. Am J Transplant 2007;7(4):941–8.
24. Wang Y, Lan GB, Peng FH, et al. Cancer risks in recipients of renal transplants: a meta-analysis of cohort studies. Oncotarget 2018;9(20):15375–85.
25. Grulich AE, van Leeuwen MT, Falster MO, et al. Incidence of cancers in people with HIV/AIDS compared with immunosuppressed transplant recipients: a meta-analysis. Lancet 2007;370(9581):59–67.
26. Maisonneuve P, Agodoa L, Gellert R, et al. Cancer in patients on dialysis for end-stage renal disease: an international collaborative study. Lancet 1999; 354(9173):93–9.
27. Engels EA, Pfeiffer RM, Fraumeni JF Jr, et al. Spectrum of cancer risk among US solid organ transplant recipients. JAMA 2011;306(17):1891–901.
28. Collett D, Mumford L, Banner NR, et al. Comparison of the incidence of malignancy in recipients of different types of organ: a UK Registry audit. Am J Transplant 2010;10(8):1889–96.
29. Krynitz B, Edgren G, Lindelöf B, et al. Risk of skin cancer and other malignancies in kidney, liver, heart and lung transplant recipients 1970 to 2008–a Swedish population-based study. Int J Cancer 2013;132(6):1429–38.
30. Tessari G, Naldi L, Boschiero L, et al. Incidence of primary and second cancers in renal transplant recipients: a multicenter cohort study. Am J Transplant 2013; 13(1):214–21.
31. Opelz G, Döhler B. Lymphomas after solid organ transplantation: a collaborative transplant study report. Am J Transplant 2004;4(2):222–30.
32. Kotton CN, Huprikar S, Kumar D. Transplant Infectious Diseases: A Review of the Scientific Registry of Transplant Recipients Published Data. Am J Transplant 2017;17(6):1439–46.
33. Sarkar M, Bramham K, Moritz MJ, et al. Reproductive health in women following abdominal organ transplant. Am J Transplant 2018;18(5):1068–76.
34. McKay DB, Josephson MA, Armenti VT, et al. Reproduction and transplantation: report on the AST Consensus Conference on Reproductive Issues and Transplantation. Am J Transplant 2005;5(7):1592–9.
35. Danziger-Isakov L, Kumar D. Vaccination of solid organ transplant candidates and recipients: Guidelines from the American society of transplantation infectious diseases community of practice. Clin Transplant 2019;33(9):e13563.

Pregnancy in Chronic Kidney Disease

Acute Kidney Injury in Pregnant Women and Management of Chronic Kidney Disease in the Pregnant Patient

Arundati Rao, MBBS[a], Ursula C. Brewster, MD[a],*

KEYWORDS

- Hypertension • Hypertensive disorders of pregnancy • Preeclampsia
- Kidney disease in pregnancy

KEY POINTS

- As women pursue pregnancy with underlying medical problems such as hypertension and kidney disease, management of these is relevant to clinical practice and requires a multidisciplinary approach.
- Hypertension in pregnancy is defined by blood pressure (BP) greater than or equal to 140/90 mm Hg. Chronic hypertension predates pregnancy, whereas gestational hypertension is characterized by elevation in BP after 20 weeks of gestation in the absence of proteinuria.
- There are several important risk factors for preeclampsia (PEC). Aspirin, 81 mg, plays a role in prevention of PEC in those at risk.
- Management of acute kidney injury, chronic kidney disease, and end-stage kidney disease in pregnancy varies from its usual management and requires a multidisciplinary team approach.
- In kidney transplant recipients, management begins with reproductive counseling, and pregnancy is advised after 1 year of transplantation, with stable allograft function, off teratogenic medications.

INTRODUCTION

In the United States, prevalence of hypertension is 45.4% and increases with age.[1] CDC estimates prevalence of chronic kidney disease (CKD) is 15% among adults and 14% among women. Diabetes and hypertension are also increasingly common among young women. As women pursue pregnancy with these conditions,

---

[a] Yale University School of Medicine, 330 Cedar Street, BB114, New Haven, CT 06510, USA
* Corresponding author.
E-mail address: ursula.brewster@yale.edu

Med Clin N Am 107 (2023) 717–726
https://doi.org/10.1016/j.mcna.2023.03.005
0025-7125/23/© 2023 Elsevier Inc. All rights reserved.

medical.theclinics.com

management of CKD and hypertension in pregnancy is becoming increasingly relevant to general clinical practice. Women will often look to their primary care providers for advice and management of these issues. Common nephrological complications including PEC, pregnancy-related acute kidney injury (p-AKI), and management of pregnancy in kidney transplant recipients are discussed in this article.

It is first important to understand the physiologic changes that are relevant to the kidney that occur during pregnancy.[2] Normally, the changes include the following:

- A decrease in systemic vascular resistance and mean arterial pressure, which manifests as a decrease in blood pressure (BP)
- A decrease in systemic vascular resistance, and decline in afterload results in an increase in cardiac output
- Increasing glomerular hyperfiltration presents as decline in serum creatinine from baseline
- Plasma volume expansion
- Dilated urinary collecting system often noted on ultrasonography

HYPERTENSION
Definitions

- According to American College of Obstetrics and Gynecology (ACOG) 2013 guidelines, hypertension in pregnancy is defined based on BP greater than or equal to 140/90 mm Hg.[3]
- Chronic hypertension is defined as hypertension that predates pregnancy, whereas gestational hypertension is characterized by elevation in BP after 20 weeks of gestation in the absence of proteinuria.
- In addition, chronic hypertension may be superimposed by development of PEC.[3]

A population-based study found that the incidence of hypertensive disorders of pregnancy and PEC is 15.3% on a per-woman basis and 7.5% on a per-pregnancy basis.[4] The study also found women with history of hypertensive disorders of pregnancy had increased risk of stroke, coronary artery disease, cardiac arrhythmias, and kidney disease.[4] Although the rates of maternal mortality have declined over time, hypertension remains one of the leading causes of mortality after abortion and hemorrhage.[5] Risks of chronic hypertension to the fetus include stillbirth, growth restriction, preterm birth, and congenital abnormalities.[6–9]

Treatment thresholds and targets for hypertensive disorders of pregnancy vary based on individual society guidelines. ACOG recommends antihypertensive therapy for all women with PEC, sustained systolic BP (SBP) greater than or equal to 160 mm Hg or diastolic BP (DBP) greater than or equal to 110 mm Hg, and chronic hypertension with SBP greater than or equal to 140 mm Hg and DBP greater than or equal to 90 mm Hg. ACOG defines target BP between 120 and 160/80 to 110 mm Hg.[10] Drugs safe in pregnancy are outlined in **Table 1**.

Use of renin-angiotensin-aldosterone blocking agents is contraindicated in pregnancy, and diuretics such as hydrochlorothiazide should only be used in very rare circumstances after conferring with the obstetrician.

CLINICS CARE POINTS

- Although the American College of Cardiology/American Heart Association diagnostic criteria for hypertension in adults has recently changed, ACOG defines hypertension in pregnancy based on BP greater than or equal to 140/90 mm Hg.

Table 1
Hypertension drugs commonly used in pregnancy[10]

Medication Name	Drug Class	Dose	Notes
Alpha methyldopa	Alpha-2-antagonists	500–3000 mg/d PO in 2–4 divided doses	Can cause sedation, depression, dizziness
Labetalol	Beta-blockers	200–2400 mg/d PO in 2–3 divided doses	Avoid in patients with asthma, decompensated heart failure, bradycardia. Metoprolol as alternative if labetalol not available. Atenolol is NOT recommended due to risk of growth restriction and low birth weight.
Nifedipine	Calcium channel blockers	30–120 mg/d PO once daily extended-release formulation	Amlodipine is considered safe based on small studies. Immediate release can be used in acute severe hypertension.
Hydralazine	Vasodilators	5–10 mg IV, max 20 mg	Used in acute severe hypertension. Limited by reflex tachycardia, hypotension, headaches, and so forth

Abbreviation: IV, intravenous.

- Chronic hypertension predates the onset of pregnancy, and gestational hypertension is diagnosed AFTER 20 weeks of gestation in the absence of proteinuria.
- ACOG recommends antihypertensive therapy for all women with PEC, sustained SBP greater than or equal to 160 mm Hg or DBP greater than or equal to 110 mm Hg, and chronic hypertension with SBP greater than or equal to 140 mm Hg and DBP greater than or equal to 90 mm Hg.
- Drugs commonly used for hypertension management in pregnancy include labetalol and nifedipine, whereas intravenous labetalol, hydralazine, and short-acting nifedipine are used to manage acute severe hypertension.
- Renin-angiotensin-aldosterone system (RAAS) inhibitors are contraindicated in pregnancy.

PREECLAMPSIA

PEC is defined by hypertension and proteinuria or in the absence of proteinuria, any of the following: thrombocytopenia (platelets < 100,000/μL), abnormal liver function tests, new-onset worsening kidney function, pulmonary edema, or cerebral disturbance.[3]

From pathophysiologic standpoint, PEC begins with abnormal placentation during the first trimester, characterized by inadequate remodeling of maternal uterine spiral arterioles resulting in relative placental ischemia.[11] Later in pregnancy, elevated levels of soluble fms-like tyrosine kinase 1 (sFLT1) and soluble endoglin (sENG), circulating antiangiogenic factors, typifies PEC. sFLT1 and sENG antagonize vascular endothelial growth factor and transforming growth factor β signaling, which leads to development of endothelial dysfunction and ultimately, hypertension, proteinuria, and glomerular endotheliosis.[12,13] Other factors involved in the pathogenesis of PEC include proinflammatory cytokines, complement dysregulation, and alterations in RAAS and sympathetic nervous system, which are elegantly reviewed by Rana and colleagues.[14]

Other risk factors include nulliparity, systemic lupus erythematosus, prepregnancy BMI greater than or equal to 25 kg/m^2, advanced maternal age greater than 35 years, antiphospholipid syndrome, and assisted reproductive technologies (**Box 1**).[15]

Definitive management of PEC is timely delivery; however, components of management begin with preconception counseling and extend to management of short-term and long-term complications. Prenatal aspirin therapy plays an important role in prevention of PEC in high-risk patients. All at-risk women should be started on 81 mg of aspirin daily at the beginning of the second trimester as an effective preventative strategy. Treatment and close monitoring of blood pressures and identifying other high-risk features is important in ensuring safe maternal and fetal outcomes. In the peripartum period, there is increased risk of peripartum cardiomyopathy and its related complications. Long-term complications are listed in **Box 2**.

Box 1
Strong risk factors for preeclampsia[15]

Prior preeclampsia

Chronic hypertension

Prepregnancy body mass index greater than or equal to 30

Diabetes mellitus

Chronic kidney disease

Box 2
Long-term complications of preeclampsia[16–18]

Hypertension

Cardiovascular disease (CVD)

Cerebrovascular disease

Peripheral arterial disease

Cardiovascular mortality

End-stage kidney disease (ESKD)

Cardiovascular disease in children born to preeclamptic mother

---

CLINICS CARE POINTS

- PEC is defined by hypertension and proteinuria or in the absence of proteinuria, any of the following: thrombocytopenia (platelets < 100,000/μL), abnormal liver function tests, new-onset worsening kidney function, pulmonary edema, or cerebral disturbance.

- Management of PEC includes prevention with low-dose aspirin in high-risk patients, treatment of hypertension, and monitoring for complications. Definitive treatment is timely delivery.

- PEC is associated with short-term complications including peripartum cardiomyopathy and long-term complications, particularly cardiovascular disease (CVD) and ESKD, in the mother and CVD in children born to preeclamptic mothers.

KIDNEY DISEASE IN PREGNANCY

Normal pregnancy is associated with the following physiologic kidney changes[2]:

- As mentioned previously, glomerular filtration rate increases, which presents clinically as decline in serum creatinine; this means that a "normal" serum creatinine in a pregnant patient may indicate compromised kidney function.
- Altered tubular function with increase in mild proteinuria, variable change in glycosuria.
- Hyponatremia due to increased total body water
- Anatomically, dilation of the collecting system, which presents as mild hydronephrosis on imaging.

Acute Kidney Injury and Pregnancy

p-AKI is associated with increased maternal and fetal morbidity and mortality.[19] The landscape of p-AKI has evolved over time, and there is increased incidence of p-AKI in the developed world attributed to advanced maternal age, hypertensive disorders of pregnancy, and underlying CKD.[20] The causes of p-AKI are broad. And unlike in the general population where the differential diagnosis of AKI is divided into prerenal, intrarenal, and postrenal causes, in pregnancy the differential diagnosis should be organized based on gestational age, which is summarized in **Table 2**.

Management of p-AKI begins with diagnosis, which can be challenging. History, physical examination, appropriate laboratory testing, and imaging are initial strategies. Kidney biopsy may be indicated to define underlying intrinsic pathology when a diagnosis is not clear from alternative information but this should only be done in the first

Table 2
Causes of acute kidney injury in pregnancy[21,22]

Before 20 wk	After 20 wk	Any Time
Volume Depletion from hyperemesis gravidarum	Preeclampsia/Eclampsia	Hypotension (hypovolemia, cardiomyopathy, sepsis)
Septic abortion	Hemolysis, elevated liver enzymes, low platelet count (HELLP) syndrome	Undiagnosed CKD
—	Hemolytic uremic syndrome (HUS)	Pyelonephritis
—	Thrombotic thrombocytopenic purpura (TTP)	Medication related
—	Acute fatty liver disease of pregnancy	—
—	Placental abruption or hemorrhage	—
—	Obstructive uropathy	—

20 weeks unless absolutely necessary. Risk of kidney biopsy increases in the latter half of pregnancy.

Ultimately, treatment is based on the underlying cause and may include delivery of fetus and dialysis. Management of p-AKI should involve a multidisciplinary approach including obstetrics, nephrology, neonatology.

Chronic Kidney Disease and Pregnancy

Four percent of women in child-bearing age have CKD.[23] Advanced CKD is associated with higher rates of infertility and early pregnancy loss. When pregnancy occurs in women with CKD, it associated with adverse outcomes in maternal and fetal health. Importantly, pregnancy itself is a risk factor for accelerated progression of CKD, which is important to discuss in preconceptive counseling with your patients.[23] Adverse maternal and fetal events are detailed in **Table 3** and occur more frequently with higher stage of baseline CKD.[23]

End-Stage Kidney Disease and Pregnancy

Dialysis patients of reproductive age frequently have irregular menstrual cycles and infertility. The diagnosis of pregnancy can be challenging as beta-human chorionic gonadotrophin (B-HCG) is renally cleared, so can be elevated even in nonpregnant

Table 3
Adverse outcomes in patients with chronic kidney disease and pregnancy

Maternal Adverse Outcomes	Fetal Adverse Outcomes
Worsening hypertension	Prematurity
Proteinuria	Low birth weight
Preeclampsia	Fetal loss
HELLP syndrome	—
Decline in kidney function	—

Abbreviation: HELLP, hemolysis, elevated liver enzymes, low platelet count.

patients. For that reason, pregnancy is confirmed by serum B-HCG measurements combined with diagnostic ultrasound. Pregnancy in patients with ESKD is associated with adverse maternal and fetal outcomes compared with the general population. A study comparing outcomes between 2 cohorts, one from Canada (N = 22) and one from United States (N = 70), showed a dose response between dialysis intensity and pregnancy outcomes.[24] Outcome of the study was higher live birth rate in women dialyzed greater than 36 hours per week. These data support the practice of dialyzing pregnant patients at least 36 hours per week.

CLINICS CARE POINTS

- The physiologic responses to pregnancy include glomerular hyperfiltration with lower serum creatinine, mild increase in proteinuria, increase in total body sodium and potassium with lower serum levels of both, and dilation of the collecting system.
- Incidence of p-AKI has increased in developed countries, is associated with adverse maternal and fetal outcomes, and its management is based on underlying cause and associated complications.
- CKD is associated with lower fertility and if pregnancy occurs, may be associated with adverse maternal and fetal outcomes including pregnancy loss.
- Patients of reproductive age on dialysis may become pregnant, and outcomes of pregnancy improve with intensive dialysis regimens.

KIDNEY TRANSPLANT AND PREGNANCY

Counseling regarding pregnancy is key in the pretransplant and posttransplant period. Discussion topics must include fertility, contraception, timing of pregnancy, allograft outcomes following pregnancy, and so forth.

In patients on dialysis, pregnancy rates are low; however, fertility may return following kidney transplantation (KT) in some women. A study by Saha and colleagues evaluated the dysfunction of the hypothalamic-pituitary-gonadal axis that occurs in patients with chronic kidney disease and changes that occur following transplantation. The results suggest normalization of the axis by about 6 months following KT.[25]

American Society of Transplantation Consensus Conference on Reproductive Issues and Transplantation from 2005 recommended patients of reproductive age to undergo counseling on contraception before KT to determine the optimal choice based on risks and benefits, cost, and so forth.[26] Although barrier methods are commonly recommended, they are the least effective of current options. Progestin-only pills were reported to not be associated with adverse side effects. Drug interactions between immunosuppression (IS) and contraceptives must be considered.

In general, for the best pregnancy outcomes, it is recommended to wait 1 year posttransplantation, have stable allograft function without evidence of proteinuria, well-controlled comorbidities (eg, hypertension, diabetes mellitus, and so forth), or low risk of opportunistic infection (eg, cytomegalovirus), and be off teratogenic medications (eg, mycophenolic acid).[26]

Drugs considered safe in pregnancy include corticosteroids, calcineurin inhibitors (eg, tacrolimus), and azathioprine. On the other hand, mycophenolic acid is teratogenic and would be discontinued before conception. A table with detailed adverse effects on maternal and fetal health may be found in this review by Chandra and colleagues.[27]

Patients who successfully become pregnant must be managed by a multidisciplinary team including transplant physicians and obstetricians. The goals of the team include maternal well-being and health including stability of allograft function, as well as optimal fetal growth. These patients are closely monitored for blood pressure control, allograft function, adequacy of IS, and so forth.

Pregnancy risks include PEC, preterm delivery, and low birth weight.[28] Although allograft loss due to rejection is a concern, current IS strategies have lowered rates of rejection in general. Patients with a recent episode of rejection or serum creatinine greater than 1.5 mg/dL are considered to have high risk.[26]

Breastfeeding in KT recipients on IS has not been well studied and is controversial. Although there is no definitive recommendation on breastfeeding, it is not absolutely contraindicated.[26]

CLINICS CARE POINTS

- Counseling patients pretransplantation and posttransplantation on fertility, contraception, and pregnancy is paramount.
- Multidisciplinary approach is required to care for a pregnant kidney transplant recipient and must include transplant physicians and high-risk obstetricians.
- Assessment includes medication review, monitoring of allograft function, blood pressure, fetal growth, and so on.

SUMMARY

Pregnancy in women with CKD presents unique challenges for mom and provider but can be safely undertaken with proper supervision. Preconceptive counseling is an essential part of the care plan and should involve primary providers, obstetricians, and nephrologists. Normal physiologic changes in pregnancy may affect blood pressure and proteinuria measurements. Blood pressure must be carefully monitored and treated with medications that are safe in pregnancy. These women are at high risk for PEC and should be offered aspirin after the first trimester to lessen the risk and monitored closely. Women who are on dialysis or who have a working kidney transplant require special expertise but can be managed to successful outcome. Preterm delivery is common in these groups and should be planned for.

DISCLOSURE

The authors have no relevant financial or commercial conflicts of interest.

REFERENCES

1. Ostchega Y, Fryar CD, Nwankwo T, et al. Hypertension prevalence among adults aged 18 and over: United States, 2017-2018. NCHS Data Brief 2020;(364):1–8.
2. Odutayo A, Hladunewich M. Obstetric nephrology: renal hemodynamic and metabolic physiology in normal pregnancy. Clin J Am Soc Nephrol 2012;7(12): 2073–80.
3. Hypertension in pregnancy. Report of the American College of Obstetricians and Gynecologists' Task Force on Hypertension in Pregnancy. Obstet Gynecol 2013; 122(5):1122–31.
4. Garovic VD, White WM, Vaughan L, et al. Incidence and long-term outcomes of hypertensive disorders of pregnancy. J Am Coll Cardiol 2020;75(18):2323–34.

5. Kassebaum NJ, Bertozzi-Villa A, Coggeshall MS, et al. Global, regional, and national levels and causes of maternal mortality during 1990-2013: a systematic analysis for the Global Burden of Disease Study 2013. Lancet 2014;384(9947): 980–1004.

6. Jain L. Effect of pregnancy-induced and chronic hypertension on pregnancy outcome. J Perinatol 1997;17(6):425–7.

7. Panaitescu AM, Baschat AA, Akolekar R, et al. Association of chronic hypertension with birth of small-for-gestational-age neonate. Ultrasound Obstet Gynecol 2017;50(3):361–6.

8. Panaitescu AM, Syngelaki A, Prodan N, et al. Chronic hypertension and adverse pregnancy outcome: a cohort study. Ultrasound Obstet Gynecol 2017;50(2): 228–35.

9. Ramakrishnan A, Lee LJ, Mitchell LE, et al. Maternal hypertension during pregnancy and the risk of congenital heart defects in offspring: a systematic review and meta-analysis. Pediatr Cardiol 2015;36(7):1442–51.

10. American College of Obstetricians and Gynecologists' Committee on Practice Bulletins—Obstetrics. ACOG Practice Bulletin No. 203: Chronic Hypertension in Pregnancy. Obstet Gynecol 2019;133(1):e26–50.

11. Zhou Y, Damsky CH, Fisher SJ. Preeclampsia is associated with failure of human cytotrophoblasts to mimic a vascular adhesion phenotype. One cause of defective endovascular invasion in this syndrome? J Clin Invest 1997;99(9):2152–64.

12. Maynard SE, Min JY, Merchan J, et al. Excess placental soluble fms-like tyrosine kinase 1 (sFlt1) may contribute to endothelial dysfunction, hypertension, and proteinuria in preeclampsia. J Clin Invest 2003;111(5):649–58.

13. Venkatesha S, Toporsian M, Lam C, et al. Soluble endoglin contributes to the pathogenesis of preeclampsia. Nat Med 2006;12(6):642–9.

14. Rana S, Lemoine E, Granger JP, et al. Preeclampsia: pathophysiology, challenges, and perspectives. Circ Res 2019;124(7):1094–112.

15. Bartsch E, Medcalf KE, Park AL, et al. Clinical risk factors for pre-eclampsia determined in early pregnancy: systematic review and meta-analysis of large cohort studies. BMJ 2016;353:i1753.

16. McDonald SD, Malinowski A, Zhou Q, et al. Cardiovascular sequelae of pre-eclampsia/eclampsia: a systematic review and meta-analyses. Am Heart J 2008;156(5):918–30.

17. Vikse BE, Irgens LM, Leivestad T, et al. Preeclampsia and the risk of end-stage renal disease. N Engl J Med 2008;359(8):800–9.

18. Davis EF, Lazdam M, Lewandowski AJ, et al. Cardiovascular risk factors in children and young adults born to preeclamptic pregnancies: a systematic review. Pediatrics 2012;129(6):e1552–61.

19. Liu Y, Ma X, Zheng J, et al. Pregnancy outcomes in patients with acute kidney injury during pregnancy: a systematic review and meta-analysis. BMC Pregnancy Childbirth 2017;17(1):235.

20. Rao S, Jim B. Acute kidney injury in pregnancy: the changing landscape for the 21st century. Kidney Int Rep 2018;3(2):247–57.

21. Piccoli GB, Zakharova E, Attini R, et al. Acute kidney injury in pregnancy: the need for higher awareness. A pragmatic review focused on what could be improved in the prevention and care of pregnancy-related AKI, in the year dedicated to women and kidney diseases. J Clin Med 2018;7(10):318.

22. Taber-Hight E, Shah S. Acute kidney injury in pregnancy. Adv Chronic Kidney Dis 2020;27(6):455–60.

23. Fischer MJ. Chronic kidney disease and pregnancy: maternal and fetal outcomes. Adv Chronic Kidney Dis 2007;14(2):132–45.

24. Hladunewich MA, Hou S, Odutayo A, et al. Intensive hemodialysis associates with improved pregnancy outcomes: a Canadian and United States cohort comparison. J Am Soc Nephrol 2014;25(5):1103–9.

25. Saha MT, Saha HH, Niskanen LK, et al. Time course of serum prolactin and sex hormones following successful renal transplantation. Nephron 2002;92(3):735–7.

26. McKay DB, Josephson MA, Armenti VT, et al. Reproduction and transplantation: report on the AST Consensus Conference on Reproductive Issues and Transplantation. Am J Transplant 2005;5(7):1592–9.

27. Chandra A, Midtvedt K, Asberg A, et al. Immunosuppression and reproductive health after kidney transplantation. Transplantation 2019;103(11):e325–33.

28. Deshpande NA, James NT, Kucirka LM, et al. Pregnancy outcomes in kidney transplant recipients: a systematic review and meta-analysis. Am J Transplant 2011;11(11):2388–404.

Nephrotic Syndrome for the Internist

Maria Jose Zabala Ramirez, MD, Eva J. Stein, MD, Koyal Jain, MD, MPH*

KEYWORDS

- Glomerulonephritis • Nephrotic syndrome • Nephrotic syndrome/complications
- Nephrotic syndrome/pathophysiology • Nephrotic syndrome/management • Edema
- Hypoalbuminemia • Proteinuria

KEY POINTS

- Nephrotic syndrome (NS) is caused by a wide range of immunologic, infectious, malignant, and metabolic etiologies.
- NS presents with the constellation of edema, proteinuria of greater than 3 to 3.5 g per day, hypoalbuminemia, and hyperlipidemia.
- The complications of NS include edema, cardiovascular disease, kidney impairment, infections, and thrombosis.
- The initial serologic evaluation and supportive management of NS should start in the primary care office. Histologic diagnosis and directed therapy should be conducted by a nephrologist.

BACKGROUND

Nephrotic syndrome (NS) is a disorder of the kidney that is defined by the presence of greater than 3 to 3.5 g per day of proteinuria, which results in hypoalbuminemia, edema, and hyperlipidemia. NS occurs due to a disruption of the glomerular filtration barrier. This specialized barrier consists of three layers: fenestrated endothelial capillary cells, a basement membrane, and epithelial cells known as podocytes. This filtration barrier selectively filters fluid and solutes while preventing passage of protein and cells (**Fig. 1**). The structure is both size- and charge-selective, favoring passage of smaller or cationic molecules over larger or anionic molecules. The physiologic size of pores through the barrier creates the size selectivity.[1] The endothelial cells are covered by a negatively charged surface layer that creates the charge selectivity.[2] The consequence of this structure is that important proteins, such as albumin, immunoglobulins, and coagulation enzymes are preserved under normal conditions. NS occurs when sufficient

Division of Nephrology and Hypertension, Department of Medicine, UNC Kidney Center, University of North Carolina at Chapel Hill, 7024 Burnett Womack Building, CB 7155, Chapel Hill, NC 27599, USA
* Corresponding author.
E-mail address: koyal_jain@med.unc.edu

Med Clin N Am 107 (2023) 727–737
https://doi.org/10.1016/j.mcna.2023.03.006
0025-7125/23/© 2023 Elsevier Inc. All rights reserved.

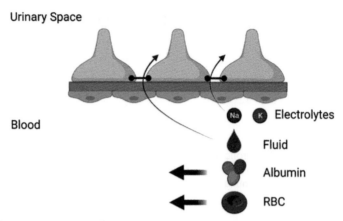

Fig. 1. Filtration barrier. The filtration barrier, which consists of three layers: fenestrated endothelial capillary cells, a basement membrane, and epithelial cells known as podocytes. As shown in this figure, this barrier selectively filters fluid and solutes and prevents the passage of protein and cells.

disruption occurs to various parts of filtration barrier, allowing for pathologic protein loss and leading to the complications described later in this article.

CAUSES OF NEPHROTIC SYNDROME

The primary classes of NS are minimal change disease, membranous nephropathy, and focal segmental glomerulosclerosis (FSGS). These classes are defined by the pattern of histologic lesions seen on a kidney biopsy. Each pattern of injury can be primary (or idiopathic), secondary to a systemic disease or exposure, or genetic, meaning that the underlying genetic abnormality has been identified. Outside of these primary causes are disease states that cause specific histologic lesions, such as amyloidosis and diabetic nephropathy. Membranoproliferative glomerulonephritis (MPGN) can present with an overlapping syndrome consisting of both nephritic and nephrotic features. **Table 1** demonstrates an overview of the common causes of NS.

COMPLICATIONS AND PATHOPHYSIOLOGY
Edema

Edema is the most defining feature of NS going back to even its earliest descriptions. Hippocrates described a state of generalized edema with the observation "when bubbles settle on the surface of the urine, it indicates a disease of the kidney and that the disease will be protracted."[3] The pathophysiology of edema in NS is primarily described by two primary theories: the "underfill" and "overfill" hypotheses.[4,5]

According to the "underfill" hypothesis, low serum albumin level caused by urinary protein losses is the primary driver of edema. Low serum albumin leads to leakage of fluid out of the vessels and into the interstitial space. This leads to low intravascular pressure and reduced renal perfusion, which stimulates the renin-angiotensin-aldosterone (RAAS) system and causes sodium retention and edema. Although physiologically appealing, this hypothesis does not seem to fully explain the edema observed in NS.[4,5]

The "overfill" hypothesis, in contrast, explains fluid retention in NS by direct changes to sodium handling by the kidneys.[4] Specifically, the changes seem to occur at the

Table 1
Classification of nephrotic syndrome by histology and common etiologies

Histology/Primary Disease	Secondary Causes (Examples)	Important Genetic Contributors
Minimal change	Drugs (NSAIDs, antibiotics, lithium, immune checkpoint inhibitors) Malignancies (hematologic) Infections (tuberculosis, HCV, Lyme disease) Allergies (bee stings, cat fur, fungi, poison ivy, ragweed pollen, dust)	
Membranous nephropathy	Lupus nephritis (class V) Drugs (NSAIDs, TNF-inhibitors, penicillamine) Infections (HBV, syphilis) Malignancies (solid tumors) Immunologic (immunoglobulin G4-related disease, graft versus host disease)	PLA2R antibody, THSD7, NELL1
FSGS	Glomerular hyperfiltration (obesity, unilateral kidney, low birth weight) Drugs (heroin, bisphosphonates, lithium, calcineurin inhibitors, anthracyclines) Infections (HIV, EBV, CMV, Parvovirus B19)	APOL1, NPHS1-2, ACTN4, TRPC6
Amyloidosis	Amyloid A amyloidosis, amyloid light chain amyloidosis	ALECT2, ATTR
MPGN	Viral infections (HBV, HCV) Autoimmune diseases (SLE, Sjogren's syndrome, rheumatoid arthritis) Cryoglobulinemia Bacterial infections (staphylococcus, streptococci, tuberculosis) Monoclonal gammopathies Fungal and parasitic infections Complement-mediated MPGN	Genetic complement abnormalities

Abbreviations: ACTN4, actinin alpha 4; ALECT2, amyloid leukocyte chemotactic factor 2; Amyloid, transthyretin; APOL1, apolipoprotein L1; CMV, cytomegalovirus; EBV, Epstein–Barr virus; NELL1, neural EGFL-like 1; NPHS1, nephrin; NPHS2, podocin; NSAIDs, nonsteroidal anti-inflammatory drugs; PLA2R, phospholipase A2 receptor; SLE, systemic lupus erythematosus. THSD7; thrombospondin, type-1 domain-containing 7A; TNF, tumor necrosis factor; TRPC6, transient receptor potential cation channel subfamily C member 6.
Data from Refs.[36–38,40–42]

level of the epithelial sodium channel (ENaC) in the nephron. This channel, when inserted into the tubular epithelium of the cortical collecting duct, allows for sodium reabsorption back into circulation. According to the "overfill" hypothesis, a primary increase in ENaC activity drives increased sodium retention. This hypothesis has been supported by rat models demonstrating increased ENaC channel expression, which seems to be triggered by the presence of proteins in the urine.[6–10] In support of this hypothesis, there are rat models and limited human data demonstrating the resolution of sodium retention in response to ENaC blockade.[11,12] In addition to primary sodium retention, there are neurohormonal changes in vasopressin and aldosterone that contribute to fluid retention in NS.[4]

Hypercoagulability

Arterial and venous thrombosis represents an important complication of NS. The underlying histopathology of NS is a significant determinant of thrombotic risk, with membranous nephropathy carrying the highest risk of thromboembolic events.[13–15] Of note, NS carries a particularly elevated risk of renal vein thrombosis, with an overall 37% prevalence identified across studies of membranous nephropathy and 28% across other histopathologies.[13] Other types of thrombosis are also observed at increased rates, including arterial clots, deep vein thrombosis, and pulmonary emboli.[14,16] The pathophysiology of hypercoagulability in NS has classically been explained by urinary protein losses that alter the balance of prothrombotic to antithrombotic proteins. Specifically, urinary loss of important anticoagulant and fibrinolytic proteins, such as antithrombin and plasminogen, contributes to dysregulation of the coagulation cascade.[16–18] Another apparent cause of hypercoagulability is increased hepatic synthesis of procoagulant factors, such as factors V and VIII.[16] It is hypothesized that hypoalbuminemia triggers the increased synthesis of these proteins by the liver with a low urinary loss due to size. The particularly high risk for renal vein thrombosis may relate to local clot formation promoted by glomerular inflammation and to glomerular hemodynamic changes in NS.[13,19]

The thrombotic risk in NS correlates with the degree of hypoalbuminemia.[14,20] This correlation reflects the urinary protein losses of albumin and anti-thrombotic proteins as well as the fact that albumin is an acute phase reactant that drops in inflammatory states. The increase in thrombotic risk seen at low serum albumin levels supports anticoagulation recommendations for NS, as discussed under the management section.

Infection

Infection risk in NS is best described in the pediatric population, in whom infections are a leading cause of morbidity and mortality. Among children, invasive bacterial infections from encapsulated organisms and gram-negative enteric organisms are the most common serious infections observed.[21–23] The infection risk is multifactorial, related to both the underlying pathophysiology and the use of immune suppressive treatments. Urinary losses of immune proteins such as immunoglobulin G and reduced function of immune cells (T cells, phagocytes) are contributors to decreased immunity.[24,25] Mainstays of treatment include steroids and cytotoxic medications which endanger patients to serious infections.

Hyperlipidemia and Cardiovascular Risks

Hyperlipidemia is a hallmark laboratory finding of NS. It has classically been explained by increased hepatic synthesis of lipoproteins triggered by hypoalbuminemia.[26] There is also evidence for decreased clearance of lipoproteins relating to changes in catabolism.[26] Hyperlipidemia contributes to, though likely does not fully explain, increased cardiovascular risk observed across NS. A population-based study of 907 patients with primary NS with matched healthy adults showed a significantly elevated risk of cardiovascular events.[27] This study demonstrated an adjusted hazard ratio of 2.58 (95% CI 1.89–3.52) for acute coronary syndrome and an adjusted hazard ratio of 3.01 (95% CI 2.16–4.19) for heart failure.[27] The increased cardiovascular risk likely reflects effects from hyperlipidemia, hypercoagulability, generalized inflammation, and kidney injury.

Kidney Injury

The spectrum of kidney impairment seen in NS is broad, encompassing acute kidney injury (AKI), chronic kidney disease (CKD), and progression to end-stage kidney disease (ESKD). Etiologies for AKI include abrupt changes in renal perfusion, acute interstitial nephritis from exposure to antibiotics and diuretics, acute tubular necrosis, and rapidly progressive glomerular injury.[28] CKD can develop from recurrent AKI, treatments such as calcineurin inhibitors (CNIs), and primary glomerular injury. Rates of progression to ESKD are broadly variable based on the underlying histopathology and treatment course. The risk of progression to ESKD is highest among patients with FSGS, followed by membranous nephropathy and then minimal change disease.[27]

MANAGEMENT

Often the diagnosis of NS occurs in the primary care setting. Once diagnosed, the patient should be evaluated by a nephrologist for further management. A kidney biopsy is commonly required to diagnose the cause of NS and to guide disease-specific therapy. For this review, the authors divide the management of NS into supportive and disease-specific therapy. The main goal of treatment is to get the disease under remission and avoid progression to ESKD. This involves the use of immunosuppressive agents directed by a nephrologist. However, supportive treatment should be started by the primary care physician (PCP). It is preferable to avoid immunosuppression therapy before evaluation as this could affect the diagnosis and cause unnecessary toxicity.[29]

Initial Evaluation

The evaluation of a patient with NS requires a thorough history and physical examination to assess for potential causes. It is essential to quantify the degree of proteinuria. This can be done by obtaining a 24-hour urine collection for protein quantification or a spot protein to creatinine ratio.[30] The assessment of the estimated glomerular filtration rate (eGFR) using the CKD epidemiology collaboration eGFR creatinine equation (CKD-epidemiology [EPI]) is preferred in adults.[30] The authors recommend the CKD-EPI without the race modifier equation. An evaluation of serum albumin level and lipid profile is also important. Serologic workup can be initiated by the PCP, based on the differential diagnosis (**Table 2**).

Kidney biopsy remains the gold standard for diagnosis, as it will also guide therapy and provide prognostic information. It is usually preferable to get a kidney biopsy before starting management; however, preemptive treatment can be considered in specific clinical conditions.[30]

Supportive Management

Edema
Edema represents a huge symptomatic burden for this patient population. It causes functional limitations and results in complications, as previously discussed. Loop

Table 2
Diagnostic evaluation in patients with nephrotic syndrome

Baseline assessment	History (exposure to medications and toxins, risk factors for infections, history of diabetes or other systemic disease and family history, and so forth) 24-h urine protein to creatinine and/or random urine to protein to creatinine ratio Urinalysis with microscopy Basic metabolic panel Serum albumin level Lipid panel Hemoglobin A1C
FSGS	Genetic testing (including APOL1) Infectious workup: HIV, CMV, Parvovirus b19, EBV, HCV, SARS-COV2 History of drug use: mTOR inhibitors, CNIs, heroin, lithium, interferon, NSAIDs, anabolic steroids Kidney biopsy
Minimal change disease	History of drug use: NSAIDs Kidney biopsy
Membranous nephropathy	Serologic workup: anti-PLA2R and anti-THSD7A Screening for malignancy (age appropriate) ANA Infectious workup: HBV, HCV, HIV, and treponemal infection History of drug use: NSAIDs, penicillamine. Kidney biopsy
Amyloidosis/Multiple myeloma	Serum electrophoresis with immune fixation electrophoresis and free light chain ratio.

Abbreviations: ANA, antinuclear antibody; mTOR, mammalian target of rapamycin; SARS-COV2, severe acute respiratory syndrome coronavirus 2.
  Data from Refs.[36–38,40–42]

diuretics are the preferred agents to treat edema per the most recent Kidney Disease: Improving Global Outcomes (KDIGO) guidelines 2021.[30] There is no evidence to guide the selection of diuretics and the starting dose. The authors prefer longer acting diuretics for the treatment of edema. Intravenous (IV) administration is recommended in cases of severe or refractory edema. Response to diuretics is usually measured based on the change in daily weight and urine output. Based on expert opinion, the goal weight loss is 2 to 4 pounds per day to avoid complications.[31] The dose of loop diuretics should be titrated up until desired diuretic response is achieved. In instances when loop diuretics are not sufficient, a thiazide or thiazide-like diuretic can be used to augment diuresis.[31]

Achieving an effective diuresis regimen can be challenging due to the pharmacodynamics of these medications. Loop diuretics act on the luminal side of the tubular epithelium. To have an appropriate effect, diuretics need to reach an adequate concentration inside the tubules. This can be particularly challenging in patients with NS due to diffusion of diuretic into the extracellular space, reduced concentration inside the tubules, and binding of loop diuretics to albumin in the tubular fluid.[31] Also, most patients have some degree of gut edema that limits absorption, hence the preference for IV administration or longer-acting loop diuretics with increased bioavailability.[32] In patients with severe hypoalbuminemia (<2 g/dL), the combination of albumin infusions and loop diuretics may enhance diuresis and is reasonable to consider.[31]

Lifestyle changes

Patients with proteinuria and kidney disease should be on a sodium restricted diet (<1500–2000 mg/d). The benefit of protein restriction is currently debated. Protein restriction to less than 0.8 g/kg/d does not offer any additional advantages.[29,30] KDIGO 2021 guidelines suggest that based on the kidney function and degree of proteinuria, dietary protein restriction should be considered up to 0.8 g/kg/d, with 1 g of daily protein added per gram of urinary loss. Dietary modifications and regular physical activity are recommended to normalize body mass index (BMI), reduce central obesity, and decrease cardiovascular risk factors.[30]

Hypertension

Goal systolic blood pressure (BP) is less than 120 mm Hg with angiotensin receptor blockers (ARB) or angiotensin-converting enzyme inhibitors (ACEis) as first choice.[30] ARBs and ACEi should be increased to the maximal tolerated dose. Adding a mineralocorticoid receptor antagonist has been shown to offer further improvement in lowering BP and proteinuria, although dual-RAAS blockade is avoided for control of proteinuria alone due to the risk of hyperkalemia. If hyperkalemia develops while on RAAS blockade, a potassium-wasting diuretic can be used as tolerated.[30] As previously discussed, loop diuretics should be prescribed if volume overload is present.

Proteinuria

Reducing the amount of proteinuria has been shown to reduce the progression of kidney disease. ARB and ACEi are the mainstay of treatment. These medications should be initiated even in the absence of hypertension to the maximum tolerated doses.[30]

Most recently, sodium–glucose cotransporter-2 inhibitors (SGLT2is) have gained momentum in the management of nephrosis. It is well known that SGLT2is are beneficial in treating patients with diabetes and proteinuria as well as in delaying progression of kidney disease in patient with and without proteinuria. In a comprehensive review, Zeynegpul and colleagues reviewed nine clinical studies evaluating the use of SGLT2i in a total of 592 patients with nephrotic range proteinuria.[33] Findings support a possible beneficial effect in lowering proteinuria and delaying progression of CKD in patients with nephrotic range proteinuria. However, currently, SGLT2is are not recommended for treatment of proteinuria in NS outside of diabetic nephropathy.

Anticoagulation. The risk for thromboembolic events in patients with NS is well established; however, there is no clear evidence to guide the use of prophylactic anticoagulation in this patient population.[34] Prophylactic anticoagulation should be considered if serum albumin is less than 2.0 to 2.5 g/dL with additional risk factors for thrombosis (proteinuria >10 g, BMI >35, genetic predisposition to thromboembolic events, heart failure III–IV, recent major surgery, or prolonged immobilization).[34] Prophylactic anticoagulation should be used when the risk for a thromboembolic event exceeds the estimated risk of bleeding.[30] Aspirin can be considered in patients with high risk for thromboembolism who are not a candidate for anticoagulation due to bleeding risk.[34]

The decision to start or hold prophylactic anticoagulation should be made in collaboration with a specialist. Patients should not start anticoagulation before evaluation by a nephrologist as this could delay biopsy.[30,34] However, in patients presenting with a thromboembolic event, initiation of treatment dose anticoagulation should not be delayed.[30]

Hyperlipidemia

Lipid levels should be monitored in patients with NS. Treatment of dyslipidemia should be initiated in patients with NS, particularly in those with additional cardiovascular risk factors. Statins are the first-line pharmacologic agents to be used along with lifestyle modifications. Non-statin medications can be added if statins are not tolerated or if goal is not achieved with maximally tolerated statin doses.[30] An additional benefit of statin therapy is their anti-proteinuric effect.[35]

Infections

Patients with impaired immunity should be up to date with vaccinations. Practice guidelines recommend pneumococcal, herpes zoster, and influenza vaccination for patients with NS.[30] Screening for syphilis, hepatitis C virus (HCV), hepatitis B virus (HBV), human immunodeficiency virus (HIV), and tuberculosis is suggested in clinically appropriate patients. Pneumocystis jiroveci pneumonia prophylaxis should be prescribed for patients receiving high-dose steroids and other immunosuppressive therapy.[30]

DISEASE-SPECIFIC MANAGEMENT

Disease-specific and immunosuppressive therapy should be deferred to a nephrologist. Treatment varies with the underlying histopathology and etiology. In all types of NS, secondary causes are managed by treating the underlying disease or removing the offending agent. Here, the authors briefly review possible therapeutic approaches.

Focal Segmental Glomerulosclerosis

Patients with primary FSGS and in some cases genetic FSGS require immunosuppressive therapy.[36] High-dose steroids remain the first line of treatment (Grade 1D per KDIGO 2021).[29] In patients not responding to or intolerant to steroids, a trial of CNIs is recommended (Grade 1C).[30,36] RAAS inhibition is the cornerstone of treatment to avoid progression of CKD. Thiazide diuretics and a low sodium diet may potentiate the antiproteinuric effect of RAAS inhibition.[36]

Minimal Change Disease

The management of minimal change disease in adults is composed of RAAS blockade, low sodium intake, and glucocorticoids. The optimal steroid regimen is not well-defined. High-dose glucocorticoids should not be given for more than 16 weeks. Tapering should start 2 weeks after remission is achieved.[30,37] If there are contraindications to glucocorticoids or if the patient has relapsing disease, further immunosuppressive treatment options include cyclophosphamide, CNI, mycophenolate, and rituximab.[30,37]

Membranous Nephropathy

Primary membranous nephropathy patients should be risk-stratified before receiving immunosuppressive therapy. Low-risk patients are treated with symptom management and risk modification only. Patients at moderate risk of kidney disease progression can be managed conservatively or with immunosuppression (rituximab or CNIs and glucocorticoids). For patients at high risk, immunosuppressive therapy with rituximab, cyclophosphamide and steroids, or CNIs and rituximab is recommended. Patients at very high risk for progression to ESKD are managed primarily with cyclophosphamide and steroids.[30]

Amyloid

The management of amyloidosis with renal involvement is multidisciplinary, involving hematology/oncology and nephrology. RAAS blockade should be used cautiously in patients with amyloid light chain (AL) cardiac amyloidosis due to the risk of hypotension.

Disease-targeted therapy should be directed by specialists and will vary depending on the type of amyloid.[38]

Diabetic Nephropathy

Diabetes is one of the leading causes of NS. In addition to diabetic control and lifestyle modifications, there are medications that carry significant kidney and cardiac protective effects and that decrease proteinuria in patients with diabetic nephropathy.

Patients with diabetes and proteinuria should be initiated on RAAS blockade, even in the absence of hypertension, titrated up to the highest tolerated dose. The kidney function and potassium level should be monitored 2 to 4 weeks after initiation or dose changes.[39] Increase in the serum creatinine is expected and RAAS blockade should not be stopped unless it rises by greater than 30% and there are no other causes of AKI.[39] In the case of hyperkalemia, a low-potassium diet and potassium binders can be considered before the discontinuation of the medication. Women of reproductive age should be counseled on the teratogenic effects of RAAS blockade and initiated on contraception if pregnancy is not desired.

As previously discussed, the kidney and cardiovascular protective effects of SGLT2i in patients with kidney disease and proteinuria are well-known. SGLT2is are particularly important tools in the management of type 2 diabetic nephropathy. SGLT2i should be considered in all patients with eGFR greater than 20 mL/min/1.73 m.^{2} A drop in eGFR is expected and should not be a reason to stop the medication. Given the association of these medications with normoglycemic ketoacidosis, it is reasonable to hold them during times of high stress, prolonged fasting, or critical medical illness.[39]

SUMMARY

NS is the common presentation of a wide group of diseases that cause proteinuria, hypoalbuminemia, and edema. The diagnosis of the exact cause and disease-specific treatment requires early evaluation by a nephrologist. The internist plays a critical role in detecting early workup and general management of the disease.

CLINICS CARE POINTS

- On recognition of nephrotic syndrome, the patient should be promptly referred to nephrology, but evaluation and supportive management can begin in the primary care office.
- The initial evaluation of nephrotic syndrome should include a thorough medication review, quantification of urinary protein losses, and measurement of kidney function and lipid levels.
- The initial diagnostic evaluation can include infectious serologies, age-appropriate cancer screening, and specific antibody testing as guided by the history and physical examination.
- Supportive management includes diuresis, vaccination, blood pressure control, management of cardiovascular risk factors, suppression of proteinuria, and in some cases anticoagulation.
- Histologic diagnosis and immune suppressive therapy should be directed by a nephrologist.

DISCLOSURE

K. Jain has served as the site PI for Visterra IgA phase 2 trial and Kaneka LDL Apheresis study. Remaining authors have no other disclosures.

REFERENCES

1. Zhang A, Huang S. Progress in pathogenesis of proteinuria. Int J Nephrol 2012; 2012:314251.
2. Patrakka J, Tryggvason K. Molecular make-up of the glomerular filtration barrier. Biochem Biophys Res Commun 2010;396(1):164–9.
3. Chadwick J, Mann WN. The medical works of hippocrates: a new translation from the original Greek made especially for English readers. Blackwell; 1950.
4. Siddall EC, Radhakrishnan J. The pathophysiology of edema formation in the NS. Kidney Int 2012;82(6):635–42.
5. Gupta S, Pepper RJ, Ashman N, et al. Nephrotic Syndrome: Oedema Formation and Its Treatment With Diuretics. Front Physiol 2019;9:1868.
6. de Seigneux S, Kim SW, Hemmingsen SC, et al. Increased expression but not targeting of ENaC in adrenalectomized rats with PAN-induced NS. Am J Physiol Renal Physiol 2006;291(1):F208–17.
7. Kim SW, Wang W, Nielsen J, et al. Increased expression and apical targeting of renal ENaC subunits in puromycin aminonucleoside-induced in rats. Am J Physiol Renal Physiol 2004;286(5):F922–35.
8. Audigé A, Yu ZR, Frey BM, et al. Epithelial sodium channel (ENaC) subunit mRNA and protein expression in rats with puromycin aminonucleoside-induced nephrotic syndrome. Clin Sci (Lond). 2003;104(4):389–95.
9. Passero CJ, Mueller GM, Rondon-Berrios H, et al. Plasmin activates epithelial Na+ channels by cleaving the gamma subunit. J Biol Chem 2008;283(52): 36586–91.
10. Svenningsen P, Bistrup C, Friis UG, et al. Plasmin in nephrotic urine activates the epithelial sodium channel. J Am Soc Nephrol 2009;20(2):299–310.
11. Deschênes G, Wittner M, Stefano AD, et al. Collecting duct is a site of sodium retention in PAN nephrosis: a rationale for amiloride therapy. J Am Soc Nephrol 2001;12(3):598–601.
12. Deschênes G, Guigonis V, Doucet A. Mécanismes physiologiques et moléculaires de la constitution des oedèmes au cours du syndrome néphrotique [Molecular mechanism of edema formation in nephrotic syndrome]. Arch Pediatr 2004; 11(9):1084–94.
13. Kerlin BA, Ayoob R, Smoyer WE. Epidemiology and pathophysiology of nephrotic syndrome-associated thromboembolic disease. Clin J Am Soc Nephrol 2012; 7(3):513–20.
14. Mahmoodi BK, ten Kate MK, Waanders F, et al. High absolute risks and predictors of venous and arterial thromboembolic events in patients with nephrotic syndrome: results from a large retrospective cohort study. Circulation 2008;117(2):224–30.
15. Barbour SJ, Greenwald A, Djurdjev O, et al. Disease-specific risk of venous thromboembolic events is increased in idiopathic glomerulonephritis. Kidney Int 2012;81(2):190–5.
16. Llach F. Hypercoagulability, renal vein thrombosis, and other thrombotic complications of nephrotic syndrome. Kidney Int 1985;28(3):429–39.
17. Singhal R, Brimble KS. Thromboembolic complications in the nephrotic syndrome: pathophysiology and clinical management. Thromb Res 2006;118(3):397–407.
18. Thomson C, Forbes CD, Prentice CR, et al. Changes in blood coagulation and fibrinolysis in the nephrotic syndrome. Q J Med 1974;43(171):399–407.
19. Nickolas TL, Radhakrishnan J, Appel GB. Hyperlipidemia and thrombotic complications in patients with membranous nephropathy. Semin Nephrol 2003;23(4): 406–11.

20. Kato S, Chernyavsky S, Tokita JE, et al. Relationship between proteinuria and venous thromboembolism. J Thromb Thrombolysis 2010;30(3):281–5.
21. McIntyre P, Craig JC. Prevention of serious bacterial infection in children with nephrotic syndrome. J Paediatr Child Health 1998;34(4):314–7.
22. Moorani KN, Khan KM, Ramzan A. Infections in children with nephrotic syndrome. J Coll Physicians Surg Pak 2003;13(6):337–9.
23. Tain YL, Lin G, Cher TW. Microbiological spectrum of septicemia and peritonitis in nephrotic children. Pediatr Nephrol 1999;13(9):835–7.
24. Kliegman RM, Behrman RE, Jenson HB, et al. Nelson textbook of pediatrics. 18th edition. Philadelphia: Saunders; 2007. p. 2193–4.
25. Davison AM, Cameron JS, Grunfeld JP, et al. Oxford textbook of clinical nephrology. 3rd edition. New York: Oxford University Press; 2005. p. 421.
26. Wheeler DC, Varghese Z, Moorhead JF. Hyperlipidemia in NS. Am J Nephrol 1989;9(Suppl 1):78–84.
27. Go AS, Tan TC, Chertow GM, et al. Primary Nephrotic Syndrome and Risks of ESKD, Cardiovascular Events, and Death: The Kaiser Permanente Nephrotic Syndrome Study. J Am Soc Nephrol 2021;32(9):2303–14.
28. Koomans HA. Pathophysiology of edema and acute renal failure in idiopathic nephrotic syndrome. Adv Nephrol Necker Hosp 2000;30:41–55.
29. Politano SA, Colbert GB, Hamiduzzaman N. Nephrotic Syndrome. Prim Care 2020;47(4):597–613.
30. Kidney Disease: Improving Global Outcomes (KDIGO) Glomerular Diseases Work Group. KDIGO 2021 Clinical Practice Guideline for the Management of Glomerular Diseases. Kidney Int 2021;100(4S):S1–276.
31. Brater DC. Diuretic therapy. N Engl J Med 1998;339(6):387–95.
32. Kodner C. Diagnosis and Management of Nephrotic Syndrome in Adults. Am Fam Physician 2016;93(6):479–85.
33. Kalay Z, Sahin OE, Copur S, et al. SGLT-2 inhibitors in nephrotic-range proteinuria: emerging clinical evidence. Clinical Kidney Journal 2022;16(1):52–60.
34. Gordon-Cappitelli J, Choi MJ. Prophylactic Anticoagulation in Adult Patients with Nephrotic Syndrome. Clin J Am Soc Nephrol 2020;15(1):123–5.
35. Kalaitzidis RG, Elisaf MS. The role of statins in chronic kidney disease. Am J Nephrol 2011;34(3):195–202.
36. Rosenberg AZ, Kopp JB. Focal Segmental Glomerulosclerosis. Clin J Am Soc Nephrol 2017;12(3):502–17 [published correction appears in Clin J Am Soc Nephrol. 2018 Dec 7;13(12):1889].
37. Zamora G, Pearson-Shaver AL. Minimal Change Disease. In: StatPearls [internet]. Treasure Island (FL): StatPearls Publishing; 2022.
38. Gurung R, Li T. Renal Amyloidosis: Presentation, Diagnosis, and Management. Am J Med 2022;135(Suppl 1):S38–43.
39. Kidney Disease: Improving Global Outcomes (KDIGO) Diabetes Work Group. KDIGO 2022 Clinical Practice Guideline for Diabetes Management in Chronic Kidney Disease. Kidney Int 2022;102(5S):S1–127.
40. Alsharhan L, Beck LH Jr. Membranous Nephropathy: Core Curriculum 2021. Am J Kidney Dis 2021;77(3):440–53.
41. D'Agati VD, Kaskel FJ, Falk RJ. Focal segmental glomerulosclerosis. N Engl J Med 2011;365(25):2398–411.
42. Sethi S, Fervenza FC. Membranoproliferative glomerulonephritis–a new look at an old entity. N Engl J Med 2012;366(12):1119–31.

Secondary Hypertension Overview and Workup for the Primary Care Physician

Jeffrey M. Turner, MD[a,*], Mikhail Dmitriev, MD[b]

KEYWORDS

- Secondary hypertension • Renovascular hypertension • Primary hyperaldosteronism
- Catecholamine-secreting tumors • Coarctation of the aorta

KEY POINTS

- Secondary hypertension refers to a specific identifiable pathology leading to elevated blood pressure.
- Secondary hypertension occurs in 5%-10% of all patients diagnosed with hypertension.
- Patients should be screened for secondary hypertension if they meet the following criteria: those who have hypertension and are young in age (<30 years old), have resistant hypertension, have a sudden worsening of previously stable hypertension, present with malignant hypertension, or who have clinical characteristics suggestive of a secondary hypertension cause.
- Causes for secondary hypertension include abnormalities involving kidney function, endocrine disorders, cardiovascular abnormalities, exposure to certain drugs and substances, and monogenic inherited etiologies.
- Treatment for secondary hypertension is specific to the underlying cause and includes various strategies such as medical management, percutaneous interventions, surgery, and device therapy.

INTRODUCTION

Hypertension is a highly prevalent disease that affects 30% of US adults with annual costs of $45 billion.[1] In the overwhelming majority of patients, the cause of hypertension is multifactorial and includes aging, unhealthy lifestyle, polygenic inherited causes, as well as other factors. This is referred to as primary hypertension. However, in a small proportion of subjects, approximately 5%-10% of those with hypertension, there will exist a discrete identifiable secondary cause. Since it would not be cost-effective

[a] Section of Nephrology, Yale University School of Medicine, 330 Cedar Street, BB114, New Haven, CT 06510, USA; [b] Department of Internal Medicine, Connecticut Institute for Communities (Danbury Hospital), Danbury, CT, USA
* Corresponding author.
E-mail address: jeffrey.turner@yale.edu

Med Clin N Am 107 (2023) 739–747
https://doi.org/10.1016/j.mcna.2023.03.010
0025-7125/23/© 2023 Elsevier Inc. All rights reserved.
medical.theclinics.com

to screen everybody for a secondary cause of hypertension, it's important to be selective in who is considered for screening. Causes for secondary hypertension include abnormalities involving kidney function, endocrine disorders, cardiovascular abnormalities, exposure to certain drugs and substances, and monogenic inherited etiologies (**Box 1**). It is important to use a thoughtful approach to these patients when selecting the specific diagnostic tests to pursue as well as the management of these patients.

Box 1
Causes of secondary hypertension

Medications
  Nonsteroidal Anti-inflammatories (NSAIDs)
  Calcineurin inhibitors
  Glucocorticoids
  Oral Contraceptive Pills
  VEGF Inhibitors
  Phenylephrine
  Erythropoietin stimulating agents

Lifestyle
  Illicit drug use:
    Cocaine
    Methamphetamine
  Excessive alcohol intake
  Tobacco use
  Heavy caffeine consumption
  High sodium diet
  Black licorice (made from licorice root)

Renal
  Acute kidney injury or chronic kidney disease

Vascular
  Renovascular Hypertension:
    Atherosclerosis
    Fibromuscular Dysplasia
  Coarctation of the Aorta

Endocrine
  Primary Hyperaldosteronism:
    Adrenal Adenoma
    Bilateral Adrenal Hyperplasia
  Catecholamine-Secreting Tumors:
    Pheochromocytoma
    Paraganglioma
  Cushing syndrome
  Thyroid disorders:
    Hyperthyroidism
    Hypothyroidism
  Hyperparathyroidism
  Renin secreting tumors

Inherited Causes
  Apparent mineralocorticoid excess
  Liddle Syndrome
  Glucocorticoid remedial aldosteronism
  Gordon Syndrome

Other
  Obstructive Sleep Apnea

KNOWING WHO TO SCREEN

When considering screening, it is pragmatic to use a pre-specified set of criteria to select patients with hypertension who are more likely to have a secondary cause (**Box 2**). Hypertension that presents in subjects before the age of 30 years old should be considered atypical, and these subjects should undergo a secondary work up. Additionally, patients with resistant hypertension, in which blood pressure is not at goal despite taking adequate doses of 3 anti-hypertensive drugs (one of which is a diuretic), should also undergo a secondary work up. Further testing is also appropriate in those with a sudden change in the severity of hypertension that had previously been stable, those who present with malignant hypertension, and finally those that present with clinical characteristics that are suggestive of a secondary cause.

COMMON CAUSES OF SECONDARY HYPERTENSION
Medications and Lifestyle

Before extensive testing is undertaken, a thorough history of current medications and lifestyle factors should also be taken. Commonly used over the counter medications to look for include non-steroidal anti-inflammatory drugs and decongestants. Prescription medications such as glucocorticoids, oral contraception pills, erythropoietin stimulating agents, and calcineurin inhibitors can also drive hypertension. The presence of heavy alcohol, tobacco, or caffeine consumption should be reviewed. Patients should be asked about illicit drug use, especially cocaine and methamphetamines. Finally, the diet should be reviewed, and specific attention should be given to sodium intake.

Primary Kidney Disease

Both acute and chronic kidney disease can be accompanied by severe elevations in blood pressure. Acute kidney injury (AKI) is typically apparent based on coexisting clinical findings. The sudden onset of edema can suggest an explosive nephrotic syndrome. Meanwhile, presentations with arthralgias, rashes, and hematuria can suggest a rapidly progressive glomerulonephritis (RPGN). Both settings can be notable for severe hypertension that is difficult to manage with medications. Chronic kidney disease (CKD) is also commonly associated with hypertension, but this is typically in the setting of an absence of symptoms. Laboratory testing is critical to diagnose and stage CKD, which is solely based on elevated serum creatinine or cystatin C levels, and a reduction in the glomerular filtration which is directly determined by these biomarkers. When considering CKD as the cause of secondary hypertension, the likelihood of this correlates with the severity of CKD.[2] In other words, CKD stage 4 to 5 is often a primary etiology for secondary hypertension. However, in CKD stage 3,

---

Box 2
Clinical criteria for secondary hypertension screening

Onset of hypertension at a young age (<30 years old) with no history of obesity or diabetes

Resistant hypertension ($\geq$140/90) despite optimal dosage of three antihypertensive agents, with one being a diuretic

Sudden onset of severe hypertension, that was previously normotensive or well controlled

Malignant Hypertension

Clinical characteristics suggestive of a secondary cause (eg, hypokalemia with primary hyperaldosteronism or obesity and snoring with obstructive sleep apnea)

this is less likely to be the primary driver of severe hypertension. Therefore, it's important to maintain a high level of suspicion for other causes of secondary hypertension in subjects with early CKD.

In subjects with either AKI or CKD, diuretics and agents that inhibit the renin-angiotensin-aldosterone system (RAAS) are central to managing hypertension, the latter is especially important when proteinuria is present.[3] Specific treatments for AKI should be employed to reverse it, this may include immune-modulating drugs for inflammatory RPGNs such as IgA Nephropathy, versus antibiotics to treat postinfectious glomerulonephritis. The sudden onset of severe nephrotic syndromes typically requires some form of immunosuppressive medication such as rituximab, cyclophosphamide, or prednisone.

Renovascular Hypertension

Renovascular hypertension occurs in the setting of stenosis of the renal arteries resulting in a critical reduction of blood flow.[4] This setting triggers the upregulation of the renin-angiotensin-aldosterone system and leads to direct vasoconstriction as well as sodium retention, both of which drive hypertension.

Renal artery stenosis occurs from two distinct pathologies: fibromuscular dysplasia and atherosclerotic disease. Fibromuscular dysplasia typically occurs in young patients, more often females than males. The molecular etiology that leads to the injury of the vessel wall is unknown. Classically, the renal artery has an appearance of successive areas of narrowing and dilation, what is referred to as a string of beads on renal artery angiography. These lesions typically occur in the mid to distal portion of the artery. Atherosclerotic disease of the renal arteries occurs in patients with typical risk factors such as older age, hypertension, diabetes, active smokers, and elevated lipids. The stenotic lesion from atherosclerotic disease most often occurs in the proximal area of the artery, what is called the ostia, which is the point at which the artery branches off of the aorta and where the turbulent blood flow is found.

The diagnosis of renovascular hypertension should be suspected in any patient that meets criteria for work up of a secondary cause. In a fraction of cases, a reduction in glomerular filtration rate also occurs, this is termed ischemic nephropathy, and is a result of reduced perfusion to the kidneys. Patients can have either unilateral or bilateral disease. Patients with bilateral disease are more likely to have ischemic nephropathy, and they may poorly tolerate angiotensin-converting enzyme inhibitors (ACEi) or angiotensin receptor blockers (ARB), due to the reliance on efferent arteriole vasoconstriction to preserve glomerular pressure and glomerular filtration when renal artery stenosis is present.

Diagnostic imaging is used to make the diagnosis. A doppler ultrasound of the renal arteries is often the best initial test in non-obese patients. The presence of tardus parvus waveforms, or flow velocities greater than 180 m/s support the diagnosis of critical renal artery stenosis with secondary renovascular hypertension.[5] Computed tomography (CT) scan of the renal arteries has a higher diagnostic sensitivity than doppler ultrasound, and should be considered when ultrasound results are equivocal or when a high pre-test probability exists and doppler ultrasound testing is negative. Magnetic resonance imaging (MRI) of the renal arteries can also be used, but offers no specific benefit over a CT scan other than it allows the avoidance of having to administer potentially nephrotoxic iodinated contrast.

Treatment of renovascular hypertension depends on the underlying etiology and whether anti-hypertensive therapies are successful at lowering blood pressure. In patients with fibromuscular dysplasia, balloon angioplasty without stenting is the first-line therapy. In the majority of cases, this is curative and blood pressure resolves without the need for anti-hypertensive medications. On the other hand, in renovascular hypertension from atherosclerotic disease, first-line therapy is medical management. The preferred classes of blood pressure-lowering agents that should be used are diuretics and ACEi or ARB. Multiple randomized controlled therapies have shown no benefit of balloon angioplasty with stenting over successful use of three or fewer anti-hypertensive medications.[6,7] When adequate blood pressure reduction is not achieved despite 3 medications, or when ischemic nephropathy, flash pulmonary edema, or malignant hypertension is present despite medical therapy, balloon angioplasty with the deployment of a drug-eluting stent is indicated. In complex disease, surgical revascularization is needed, but this is done in only a minority of cases.

Primary Hyperaldosteronism

Primary hyperaldosteronism results from unregulated aldosterone production within the zona glomerulosa of one or both adrenal glands. While it was once considered to be a rare disease, primary hyperaldosteronism is now recognized as one of the more common causes of secondary hypertension.[8] Often times patients will present with hypokalemia and hypertension, which should increase one's suspicion of primary hyperaldosteronism. Metabolic alkalosis is another metabolic abnormality found in patients with primary hyperaldosteronism, but this is much less common. Up to 50% of patients with primary hyperaldosteronism will present without any metabolic abnormalities, so an absence of hypokalemia or metabolic alkalosis does not rule it out. Resistant hypertension, malignant hypertension, and hypertension at a young age should all be triggers to pursue a work up.

Primary hyperaldosteronism can result from a benign adrenal adenoma (also called Conn's Syndrome), typically occurring in a single adrenal gland, or adrenal hyperplasia, which typically involves both adrenal glands. The initial test to screen for primary hyperaldosteronism is to measure a morning plasma renin activity (PRA) and plasma aldosterone concentration (PAC). A positive test should be considered when PRA is suppressed, and PAC is elevated. An aldosterone renin ratio (ARR) > 20, with a PAC > 10 ng/dL, should prompt additional confirmatory testing.[9]

While certain anti-hypertensive medications may impact the test results of ARR testing (**Table 1**), many of these drugs can still be continued despite this. An exception to this is mineralocorticoid receptor antagonists, which can lead to an elevated PRA and falsely low ARR when they are not held prior to testing. These medications should routinely be stopped.

Confirmatory testing for primary hyperaldosteronism should include the administration of either oral sodium chloride tabs or intravenous normal saline prior to repeat measurements of aldosterone levels. If aldosterone levels remain elevated despite efforts to suppress it with sodium loading, then this confirms the diagnosis of primary

Table 1	
Medications that affect aldosterone to plasma renin ratio (ARR)	
False elevation of ARR	Beta-blockers (metoprolol, atenolol)
	Central alpha-agonists (clonidine)
False suppression of ARR	Dihydropyridine calcium-channel blockers (amlodipine, diltiazem)
	Angiotensin-converting enzyme inhibitors (lisinopril, enalapril, captopril)
	Angiotensin receptor blockers (losartan, azilsartan)
	Diuretics (thiazide and loop)
	Mineralocorticoid receptor antagonist (spironolactone)[a]

[a] Should be routinely held prior to testing.

hyperaldosteronism. However, additional testing to identify the presence of an aldosterone-producing adenoma in adrenal glands versus bilateral adrenal hyperplasia is still needed, as the treatment of these two etiologies of primary hyperaldosteronism differ. This is best accomplished with adrenal imaging using either a CT scan or MRI to identify a solitary, hypodense, adrenal adenoma > 1 cm. In a patient under 35 years of age, this finding confirms unilateral adrenal adenoma, and adrenalectomy is indicated. All other situations warrant adrenal vein sampling to evaluate for elevated aldosterone production in a single gland.[10] Patients with bilateral adrenal hyperplasia will not have lateralization of aldosterone production on this test, and therefore unilateral adrenalectomy would not be a therapeutic option in those cases. In patients over the age of 35 years of age, the risk of a silent, non-functioning adrenal adenoma is increased, hence the need for adrenal vein sampling in these patients, even when a unilateral adenoma is identified on imaging. Functioning microadenomas <1 cm not picked up on imaging can sometimes be present, and adrenal vein sampling is the only method to identify this. When adrenalectomy is not an option, such as in bilateral adrenal hyperplasia or in cases of unilateral adenomas who have high surgical risk factors that make adrenalectomy a poor option, then treatment with a mineralocorticoid receptor antagonist (spironolactone or eplerenone) is the treatment of choice.

Obstructive Sleep Apnea

Obstructive sleep apnea (OSA) is another common treatable cause of hypertension. It should be suspected in patients who snore, are obese, and report daytime somnolence. Some patients can have dozens and even hundreds of apneic episodes nightly. These episodes lead to a loss of circadian blood pressure rhythms, and this is typically manifested by a loss of the normal dipping pattern during sleep time. Activation of the sympathetic nervous system during apneic episodes contributes to this. As OSA persists, this leads to sustained activation of the sympathetic nervous system which can result in resistant hypertension and progressive cardiac dysfunction.[11]

When suspected, patients should undergo polysomnography to identify whether they have OSA and to what severity based on the frequency of apneic episodes. Treatment with continuous positive airway pressure during sleep has been shown to lower systolic and diastolic blood pressure by a mean of 2.58 mm Hg and 2.01 mm Hg respectively.[12]

UNCOMMON CAUSES OF SECONDARY HYPERTENSION
Catecholamine- Secreting Tumors-Pheochromocytomas and Paragangliomas

Pheochromocytomas are neuroendocrine tumors that arise from chromaffin cells in the adrenal medulla and result in unregulated catecholamine secretion. Paragangliomas are similar to pheochromocytomas, in that they too result in secondary hypertension from increased catecholamine secretion. However, paragangliomas are differentiated by the fact that they arise from sympathetic ganglia, typically within the abdomen, but outside of the adrenal glands. While testing for these tumors occurs frequently when secondary hypertension is suspected by clinicians, pheochromocytomas, and paragangliomas are quite rare, occurring in less than 0.2% of patients with hypertension.[13]

The classic triad at presentation is episodic headaches, sweating, and tachycardia. Patients can have either sustained or paroxysmal hypertension, and in some cases, the presentation of these tumors is marked by orthostatic hypotension rather than hypertension.

Diagnostic work up for these tumors includes the measurement of catecholamines metabolites metanephrines.[14] The measurement of plasma fractionated metanephrines is a highly sensitive test that when negative, rules out catecholamine-secreting tumors. This test, however, has a high false positive rate, especially when sampling methods are not done properly (vein cannulation followed by a 30-minute delay in blood sampling). Performing a 24-hour timed urine collection of fractionated metanephrines is less likely to lead to false positive results, and in centers where proper sampling methods are difficult to obtain, it is a better test. When these biologic tests confirm the presence of elevated catecholamine release, imaging should then be performed to confirm the location of the tumor. This can be done with either a CT scan or MRI of the abdomen and pelvis. When the tumor location is identified, additional imaging need not be done. However, when high clinical suspicion for pheochromocytoma or paraganglioma exists despite negative findings on CT scan or MRI, then functional imaging with a total body nuclear scan is indicated.

Surgical resection is the cornerstone of treatment for pheochromocytomas and paragangliomas. Preoperative steps must be taken to avoid an intraoperative hypertensive crisis. This includes the administration of an alpha blocker (typically phenoxybenzamine) at least 1 week prior to surgery. A beta blocker is also administered, but initiation should occur 2 to 3 days after starting alpha-blocker therapy. Successful surgery is usually curative of hypertension and symptoms.

Cushing Syndrome

Excess cortisol production is the hallmark of Cushing syndrome. It is the result of pituitary adenomas producing ACTH, which in turn leads to unregulated cortisol production in the adrenal glands. In addition to hypertension, patients often present with the classic features of moon facies, central obesity, proximal muscle weakness, abdominal striae, a buffalo hump fat pad, and easy bruising. Patients on chronic glucocorticoid therapy can develop an iatrogenic form of Cushing syndrome, so it is important to first rule this out as a cause. Testing includes a 24-hour urine cortisol measurement, a late night salivary cortisol test, or a dexamethasone suppression test. When two of these three tests are positive, the diagnosis of Cushing syndrome is confirmed. However, when suspicion is high despite negative testing, or when only a single test is positive, patients should be further evaluated by an endocrinologist.

Coarctation of the Aorta

Coarctation of the aorta is a severe narrowing of the aorta, typically distal to the left subclavian artery. This is usually due to a congenital malformation, but acquired coarctation can be the result of severe atherosclerosis or inflammation such as in Takayasu arteritis. While it is commonly diagnosed in childhood, some cases of aortic coarctation may not be detected until adulthood as it can often be asymptomatic with undetected hypertension. Patients will have delayed or decreased femoral pulses as compared to brachial pulses. Additionally, they will have isolated hypertension of the upper extremities, with often undetectable blood pressure in the lower extremities. The diagnosis is based on evaluating blood flow in the aorta with doppler echocardiography or thoracic imaging with a CT scan or MRI. Treatment involves surgical revision of the malformed aorta.

Thyroid and Parathyroid Diseases

Both hypothyroidism and hyperthyroidism can cause hypertension. Hypothyroidism often leads to volume retention and elevations in diastolic blood pressures. On the other hand, hyperthyroidism leads to increased cardiac output and isolated systolic hypertension with a widened pulse pressure. Measurement of thyroid stimulating hormone is a sensitive screening test for these disorders. Primary hyperthyroidism should be suspected when hypertension occurs in the setting of hypercalcemia. Hypercalcemia results in vasoconstriction due to vascular smooth muscle contraction. Direct measurement of the serum parathyroid hormone confirms the diagnosis.

Inherited Causes

In patients with a family history of resistant hypertension or hypertension at a young age, inherited causes should be suspected. This includes apparent mineralocorticoid excess, which is an autosomal recessive mutation leading to deficiency of the 11-beta-hydroxysteroid dehydrogenase enzyme. In addition, Liddle syndrome is an autosomal dominant gain of function mutation leading to the overactivation of the epithelial sodium channel (ENaC) in the principle cell of the kidney. Finally, glucocorticoid remedial aldosteronism (GRA) is another autosomal dominant mutation that leads to ACTH-sensitive aldosterone production in the zona fasciculata region of the adrenal gland. Patients with GRA can present with similar clinical features as those with primary hyperaldosteronism, but less commonly have hypokalemia. The presence of a family history of hypertension is what often raises suspicion for this disorder. In patients who an inherited cause is suspected, genetic testing is readily available for these disorders through commercially available gene panels. Many of these are covered by insurance without low or modest out-of-pocket costs.

SUMMARY

Secondary hypertension occurs in a small fraction of patients with hypertension. Once patients are properly identified for having a higher pre-test probability for a secondary cause, then screening for various etiologies should commence. Evaluations for more common causes such as renovascular hypertension and primary hyperaldosteronism should be prioritized, but in patients with clinical presentations suggestive of rare catecholamine-secreting tumors or Cushing syndrome, screening should also include tests for these disorders. Treatments will vary based on the specific causes, and depending on the underlying etiology, complete versus partial resolution of hypertension will be achieved.

CLINICS CARE POINTS

- In patients with clinical criteria suggestive of secondary hypertension, testing for the more common causes of primary hyperaldosteronism, renovascular hypertension, and thyroid disorders should be done. When additional clinical history supports it, evaluations for catecholamine-secreting tumors, Cushing syndrome, obstructive sleep apnea, and inherited disorders should also be pursued.

- For patients undergoing plasma renin activity and plasma aldosterone concentration, with the exception of mineralocorticoid receptor antagonists, anti-hypertensive medications can be continued.

- Twenty 4 hour urine fractionated metanephrines is the preferred test when evaluating patients for catecholamine-secreting tumors, as it is less likely to lead to false positive results.

- Genetic testing for inherited causes should be considered in patients with a family history of complex hypertension.

DISCLOSURES

The authors have nothing to disclose.

REFERENCES

1. Heidenreich PA, Trogdon JG, Khavjou OA, et al. Forecasting the future of cardiovascular disease in the United States: a policy statement from the American Heart Association. Circulation 2011;123(8):933–44.
2. Horowitz B, Miskulin D, Zager P. Epidemiology of hypertension in CKD. Adv Chronic Kidney Dis 2015;22(2):88–95.
3. Ku E, Lee BJ, Wei J, et al. Hypertension in CKD: Core Curriculum 2019. Am J Kidney Dis 2019;74(1):120–31.
4. Dworkin LD, Cooper CJ. Clinical practice. Renal-artery stenosis. N Engl J Med 2009;361(20):1972–8.
5. Granata A, Fiorini F, Andrulli S, et al. Doppler ultrasound and renal artery stenosis: An overview. J Ultrasound 2009;12(4):133–43.
6. Investigators A, Wheatley K, Ives N, et al. Revascularization versus medical therapy for renal-artery stenosis. N Engl J Med 2009;361(20):1953–62.
7. Cooper CJ, Murphy TP, Cutlip DE, et al. Stenting and medical therapy for atherosclerotic renal-artery stenosis. N Engl J Med 2014;370(1):13–22.
8. Brown JM, Siddiqui M, Calhoun DA, et al. The Unrecognized Prevalence of Primary Aldosteronism: A Cross-sectional Study. Ann Intern Med 2020;173(1):10–20.
9. Blumenfeld JD, Sealey JE, Schlussel Y, et al. Diagnosis and treatment of primary hyperaldosteronism. Ann Intern Med 1994;121(11):877–85.
10. Rossi GP, Funder JW. Adrenal Vein Sampling Is the Preferred Method to Select Patients With Primary Aldosteronism for Adrenalectomy: Pro Side of the Argument. Hypertension 2018;71(1):5–9.
11. Konecny T, Kara T, Somers VK. Obstructive sleep apnea and hypertension: an update. Hypertension 2014;63(2):203–9.
12. Montesi SB, Edwards BA, Malhotra A, et al. The effect of continuous positive airway pressure treatment on blood pressure: a systematic review and meta-analysis of randomized controlled trials. J Clin Sleep Med 2012;8(5):587–96.
13. Stein PP, Black HR. A simplified diagnostic approach to pheochromocytoma. A review of the literature and report of one institution's experience. Medicine (Baltim) 1991;70(1):46–66.
14. Sbardella E, Grossman AB. Pheochromocytoma: An approach to diagnosis. Best Pract Res Clin Endocrinol Metab 2020;34(2):101346.

Onco-Nephrology
Kidney Disease in the Cancer Patient

Niloufarsadat Yarandi, MD, Anushree C. Shirali, MD*

KEYWORDS

- Onco-nephrology • Acute kidney injury • Chronic kidney disease • Proteinuria
- Immune-checkpoint inhibitors • Hyponatremia • Hypomagnesemia • Hypokalemia

KEY POINTS

- Patients with cancer are at risk for kidney disease from malignancy-specific or treatment-specific causes.
- Kidney disease, particularly acute kidney injury, and hyponatremia is associated with poor outcomes in cancer patients.
- Timely referral to nephrologists experienced or trained in the care of patients with cancer (onco-nephrologists) is encouraged for timely diagnosis and management.

INTRODUCTION

Kidney disease in cancer patients requires specialized evaluation for timely and accurate diagnosis. A new Nephrology subspecialty—Onco-Nephrology—focuses on managing acute kidney injury (AKI), chronic kidney disease (CKD), proteinuria, and electrolyte disorders in these patients. Evaluation by onco-nephrologists may limit treatment disruptions of anti-cancer therapies. In this review, we outline major topics in Onco-Nephrology, focusing on those syndromes of kidney disease that all physicians, including general practitioners, are likely to encounter in clinical practice.

EPIDEMIOLOGY OF KIDNEY DISEASE IN THE CANCER PATIENT

Cancer patients experience an elevated risk of kidney disease, particularly AKI. A 2011 Danish population-based study followed 37,267 patients with an incident cancer diagnosis over 5 years[1.] At 1-year post-diagnosis, the risk of all-stage AKI was 17.5%, increasing to 27% at 5 years[1] Severe AKI (defined in this study by injury or failure category of the Risk, Injury, Failure [RIFLE] criteria) rates were at 3.5% (injury) and 1.6% (failure) at 1 year[1] Malignancy-type influenced risk, with kidney cancer having the highest 1-year AKI risk at 44%, and significant risk was also seen in patients with liver

Section of Nephrology, Yale University School of Medicine, PO Box 208029, New Haven, CT 06520-8029, USA
* Corresponding author.
E-mail address: anushree.shirali@yale.edu

Med Clin N Am 107 (2023) 749–762
https://doi.org/10.1016/j.mcna.2023.03.007
0025-7125/23/© 2023 Elsevier Inc. All rights reserved.

cancer and multiple myeloma. More contemporary data that include newer anti-cancer therapies also support heightened AKI risk following a cancer diagnosis. A 2019 Canadian study on patients who were initiated on systemic anti-cancer therapies reported cumulative AKI incidences of 3.9% and 7.8% at 1 and 5 years, respectively.[2] AKI requiring dialysis rates were 0.4% (1 year) and 0.8% (5 years). The Canadian experience suggests that even in an era of improved cancer outcomes, AKI frequently impacts cancer patients. Besides cancer type, advancing age, pre-existing CKD, male sex, and pre-existing hypertension and diabetes increase AKI risk.[2]

CKD is also prevalent among cancer patients. The Renal Insufficiency and Cancer Medications (IRMA) study retrospectively evaluated 4684 cancer patients and determined estimated glomerular filtration rate (eGFR)-based staging with Cockcroft-Gault (C-G) and Modification of Diet in Renal Disease (MDRD) formulas.[3] Depending on the formula used, the prevalence of CKD was 12.02% (MDRD) or 19.8% (C-G).[3] More recently, a Romanian database of 5831 cancer patients noted 13.4% prevalence of CKD at the end of the study, compared with the 8.8% reference rate in the general population.[4]

DIAGNOSIS OF ACUTE KIDNEY INJURY IN THE CANCER PATIENT

Diagnosing AKI in cancer patients is critical because it influences overall outcomes. A large cancer center found a 12% AKI rate in 3558 hospitalized patients over 3 months. The worsening severity of AKI was associated with increased hospital length of stay and decreased survival.[5] AKI diagnosis relies on accurately measuring the loss of GFR, with creatinine as the best-accepted serum biomarker. Other sections in this series discuss measurement of GFR, including grading of AKI. In cancer patients, serum creatinine (sCr) is the most commonly used biomarker to detect AKI, however, cancer-related sarcopenia may result in lower levels of sCr independent of kidney function. Thus, small elevations of sCr in cancer patients may actually represent severe AKI. Serum Cystatin C detects AKI at earlier time points than sCr and though not yet widely adopted, it is more accurate than sCr as a biomarker for AKI.[6]

A kidney ultrasound may refine etiology of AKI by revealing hydronephrosis from the bladder outlet or ureteral compression from tumor or lymphadenopathy. Enlarged kidneys may be seen in leukemic/lymphomatic kidney infiltration.[7] Simultaneous measurement of urine albumin and urine protein may help distinguish glomerular proteinuria from tubular proteinuria or non-albumin glomerular proteinuria such as urine light chain excretion in multiple myeloma (MM).[8] Hematuria and red blood cell casts on urinalysis in addition to proteinuria support a diagnosis of glomerulonephritis but this requires kidney biopsy for confirmation. All these diagnostic modalities—imaging, urine, etc.—are important considerations in investigating kidney disease in cancer patients.

Acute Kidney Injury in the Cancer Patient

Cancer patients are susceptible to AKI for a variety of reasons. Decreased oral intake, vomiting, and diarrhea may occur as a direct cancer effect or due to cancer treatment, putting patients at risk for AKI from pre-renal causes.[7] Risk of obstruction at any portion of the genitourinary tract is always increased in patients with cancer, and this can often be missed or underappreciated on routine imaging. Neutropenia with superimposed infections may lead to sepsis-associated acute tubular injury (ATI). In addition to these, drug nephrotoxicity from anti-cancer treatment and direct malignancy-related kidney disease is important to consider. We will review several of the major types of anti-cancer treatments, with particular attention to the most commonly used agents, as well as kidney disease associated with the direct effects of cancer.

Drug Nephrotoxicity

Advances in anti-cancer therapy have improved long-term outcomes but patients are still likely to experience kidney complications of anti-cancer therapy, including AKI, CKD, proteinuria, and hypertension. All types of treatments—conventional chemotherapy, targeted therapy, and immunotherapy—have been associated with these manifestations of kidney injury (**Table 1**).[9,10]

Conventional chemotherapy

Conventional chemotherapy is the foundational treatment of many cancers. These agents can cause both AKI and CKD via affecting vascular, interstitial, tubular, or glomerular compartments within the kidney.[11,12]

Platinum-based agents

Cisplatin, carboplatin, and oxaliplatin are alkylating agents that bind to and cross-link DNA ultimately resulting in cell death. These agents are used for treating the following malignancies: head and neck, small cell lung, ovarian, bladder, cervical, testicular, advanced urothelial, and gastrointestinal malignancies such as esophageal, colorectal, and cholangiocarcinoma.[12]

Among platinum-based agents, cisplatin has the highest rate of nephrotoxicity at 30%, followed by carboplatin at 15%, with oxaliplatin having the least nephrotoxicity at less than 5%.[12] Kidney injury with cisplatin results from direct tubular cell injury, often involving the transport cells of the proximal tubule, as well as vasoconstriction.[13] Fanconi syndrome can also occur with cisplatin exposure, and it is defined as the loss of significant electrolytes, amino acids, and other molecules in the urine due to widespread dysfunction of the transport capability within the proximal tubule of the nephron. Cisplatin-induced AKI is usually dose-, duration-, and frequency-dependent, and therefore, kidney injury typically occurs after multiple doses.[14] However, AKI has been reported after a single exposure to cisplatin.[12,15]

Methotrexate

Methotrexate (MTX) is an antimetabolite that inhibits dihydrofolate reductase to interfere with deoxyribonucleic acid (DNA) synthesis and cell replication.[12] MTX-associated AKI occurs in 3% to 60% of patients receiving high-dose MTX, which is used for central nervous system (CNS) prophylaxis in high-risk lymphoma and primary CNS lymphoma.[16] MTX nephrotoxicity results from afferent arteriolar constriction, intratubular crystal deposition, and inflammatory interstitial injury.[12] More than 80% of methotrexate and its active metabolites undergo kidney elimination, mainly by glomerular filtration and less so by tubular secretion.[17]

Aggressive IV hydration, urinary alkalinization, and folinic acid (leucovorin) are used for prevention. High-dose leucovorin along with glucarpidase and hemodialysis may be required along with above-mentioned methods in the setting of AKI and severe MTX toxicity.[12]

Ifosfamide

Ifosfamide is an alkylating agent often used with cisplatin and in the treatment of sarcomas, testicular tumors, and certain refractory lymphomas. Chloroacetaldehyde is the nephrotoxic metabolite of Ifosfamide. Ifosfamide-induced tubulointerstitial injury results in AKI from ATI or progressive CKD.[18] Proximal tubular injury may also cause complete or incomplete Fanconi syndrome, or rarely, hypokalemic, distal renal tubular

Table 1
Kidney-specific toxicity of anti-cancer therapies

	Drug Name	Nephrotoxicity	Prevention/Management
Conventional Chemotherapy	Platinum-based agents (Cisplatin, Carboplatin, Oxaliplatin)	AKI, Fanconi syndrome, dRTA, TMA, salt wasting, hypomagnesemia, mild proteinuria, polyuria, CKD, hypokalemia[12]	IV hydration, electrolyte replacement, mannitol[12]
	Methotrexate	Crystal nephropathy, inflammatory interstitial injury, afferent arteriole constriction[12]	DC NSAIDs, probenecid, penicillin, IV hydration, urinary alkalinization, Leucovorin, glucarpidase, dialysis[12]
	Pemetrexed	ATI, interstitial fibrosis, NDI, dRTA[12]	Eliminating nephrotoxins, Folic acid, B12, Hydration Kidney injury might not be reversible[12]
	Ifosfamide	Proximal tubulopathy, ATI, hemorrhagic cystitis[12]	Management: IV hydration, mesna for hemorrhagic cystitis[12]
	Gemcitabine	TMA[12]	DC gemcitabine, hemodialysis, eculizumab[12]
Targeted Therapy	BRAF/MEK inhibitors (vemurafenib, dabrafenib)	Allergic interstitial disease, ATI, Fanconi syndrome, hypophosphatemia, hypomagnesemia, hypokalemia, and sub-nephrotic-range proteinuria[34]	Monitor kidney function and electrolytes routinely, DC the agent or reduce the dose[34]
	VEGFi/TKIs (bevacizumab, ramucirumab, sunitinib, sorafenib, axitinib, pazopanib)	HTN, TMA, proteinuria[17]	Optimize BP before initiation, ACEi/ARB, CCB, discontinue the agents when indicated[17,18]
	CDK4/6 inhibitors (abemaciclib, palbociclib, ribociclib)	Pseudo-AKI, ATI[19,20]	Continue the agent after confirming pseudo-AKI[19]

| Immunotherapy | ICI (CTLA-4 inhibitor: Ipilimumab, tremelimumab; PD-1 inhibitors: Pembrolizumab, cemiplimab, nivolumab; PDL-1 inhibitor: atezolizumab, avelumab, durvalumab) | AIN, ATN, MCD, MN, lupus nephritis, pauci-immune GN, IgA nephropathy, C3 GN, FSGS, renal vasculitis, hyponatremia due to SIAD[9,21] | UA, proteinuria quantification, kidney biopsy, corticosteroids, potentially rechallenge with ICIs[21] |
| | CAR-T Therapy | Ischemic injury, hyperinflammatory state, hyponatremia due to SIADH[9,25] | Renal replacement therapy in severe cases[25] |

Abbreviations: AIN, acute interstitial nephritis; AKI, acute kidney injury; ATN, acute tubular necrosis; BRAF, v-Raf murine sarcoma viral oncogene homolog B; CAR-T, chimeric antigen receptor T-cell; CDK, cyclin-dependent kinase; CKD, chronic kidney disease; DC, discontinue; dRTA, distal renal tubular acidosis; FSGS, focal segmental glomerulosclerosis; GN, glomerulonephritis; ICI, immune-checkpoint inhibitor; IV, intravenous; MCD, minimal change disease; MEK, mitogen-activated protein kinases; MN, membranous nephropathy; NDI, nephrogenic diabetes insipidus; NSAIDs, non-steroidal anti-inflammatory drugs; SIAD, syndrome of inappropriate anti-diuretic hormone; TKI, tyrosine kinase inhibitors; UA, urinalysis; VEGFi, vascular endothelial growth factor pathway inhibitors.

acidosis, or nephrogenic diabetic insipidus. Mitochondrial dysfunction plays an important role in tubular injury pathogenesis.[18] There are limited preventive measures available for ifosfamide-induced kidney injury. Hemorrhagic cystitis due to ifosfamide can be prevented by hydration and sodium 2-mercaptoethane sulfonate (mesna).[12]

Targeted Therapies

Vascular endothelial growth factor pathway inhibitors/tyrosine kinase inhibitors
Examples of vascular endothelial growth factor pathway inhibitors (VEGFi) include bevacizumab (antibody against VEGF ligand) and ramucirumab (antibody against VEGF receptor). Tyrosine kinase inhibitors (TKI) examples are pazopanib, sorafenib, sunitinib, and axitinib, pazopanib. Both classes of agents interrupt tumor angiogenesis by inhibiting VEGF pathways and are used against renal cell carcinoma, colorectal cancer, and various other cancers. Proteinuria and hypertension are the most common adverse events. VEGFi may cause hypertension by altering sodium homeostasis or endothelial dysfunction.[19] VEGFi also may cause renal-limited thrombotic microangiopathy (TMA) manifesting as new-onset hypertension and/or proteinuria. VEGF-TKIs can cause various forms of injury to podocyte cells in the glomerulus, also known as podocytopathies. For hypertension with or without proteinuria, angiotensin-converting enzyme inhibitors (ACEIs) and angiotensin receptor blockers (ARBs) are optimal first-line treatments. In hypertension (HTN) without proteinuria, calcium channel blockers (CCBs) or ACEIs/ARBs may be used. TMA, malignant hypertension, or nephrotic-range proteinuria compel discontinuation of VEGFi.[20]

Cyclin-dependent kinase 4/6 inhibitors
Cyclin-dependent kinase (CDK) 4/6 inhibitors such as ribociclib, abemaciclib, and palbociclib are used in the treatment of certain advanced or metastatic breast cancer. These agents are associated with AKI and pseudo-AKI, which is a transient and reversible rise in serum creatinine without a change in GFR. Cr has active tubular secretion by multiple solute carrier transporters in the proximal tubular cells of the kidney and inhibition of these tubular secretory transporters by CDK 4/6 inhibitors results in decreased creatinine clearance and therefore increase in serum Cr without a true change in kidney function and GFR. Kidney-biopsy-proven ATI has been reported with these agents as well. When pseudo-AKI is clinically suspected, additional methods would reflect true kidney function more accurately in these cases, such as cystatin C.[9,21,22] Measuring iothalamate or iohexol clearances are additional methods to validate GFR values when pseudo-AKI is suspected, but these are typically available in research settings.

Immunotherapies

Immune checkpoint inhibitors
Immune checkpoint inhibitors (ICIs) are monoclonal antibodies (mAbs) that enhance tumor-directed immune responses by blocking "immune checkpoints" that downregulate the immune system. ICIs include mAbs against cytotoxic T-lymphocyte–associated antigen 4 (CTLA-4) and programmed death 1 pathway (PD-1/PD-ligand-1 [PD-L1]) and have improved outcomes in several cancers.

Increased immune system activity as a result of ICIs can cause immune-related adverse events (iRAEs). The gastrointestinal tract, skin, and endocrine system are most commonly affected. Kidney-related adverse events can occur in up to 5% of patients, especially when ICIs are used in combination with other anti-cancer therapies. AKI from acute interstitial nephritis (AIN) is the most common kidney-related iRAEs but other kidney injuries have been reported as well.[23] Reduced estimated glomerular filtration rate (eGFR), proton pump inhibitor (PPI) use and other extra-renal iRAEs are major risk factors.[24] Baseline laboratory workup including urine analysis should be obtained in patients started on ICIs. Proteinuria should be quantified if present.[23]

Chimeric antigen receptor T-cell therapy

Chimeric antigen receptor T-cell (CAR-T) therapy is novel immunotherapy consisting of reprogrammed T-cells against certain antigens in cancer cells. It may induce long-lasting remission in refractory or relapsed hematologic malignancies but is associated with significant treatment-related toxicities with multi-organ involvement.[25] In a recent study of 83 patients with resistant non-hodgkin lymphoma (NHL) receiving CAR-T, 17% developed AKI during follow-up and 71% of AKIs had resolved within 1 month of CAR-T infusion.[25]

Malignancy-Related Kidney Disease

Tumor lysis syndrome

Tumor lysis syndrome (TLS) is a medical emergency occurring in high-tumor burden malignancies. TLS may happen spontaneously but usually results following chemotherapy. Leukemia, high-grade lymphoma, and rapidly growing tumors are at high risk.[26,27]

During TLS, intracellular contents are released into the bloodstream resulting in characteristic findings of hyperkalemia, hyperuricemia, hyperphosphatemia, and hypocalcemia which can result in kidney injury, cardiac arrhythmias, seizure, and death due to multi-organ failure.[26]

Calcium phosphate, uric acid, and xanthine deposition in kidney tubules may cause crystal nephropathy. Recently, endothelial dysfunction as a result of high extra-cellular histone levels has been proposed as a crystal-independent mechanism for AKI.[27]

Management includes aggressive hydration to increase urine output to at least 2 mL per kilogram per hour and reducing uric acid by allopurinol or rasburicase. Urine alkalinization can cause calcium phosphate precipitation and is not recommended. Some patients may require renal replacement therapy due to severe AKI.[26]

Glomerular disease associated with malignancies

These glomerular diseases might occur in association with solid or hematologic malignancies and can be diagnosed even before cancer diagnosis. These glomerular diseases are heterogeneous including membranous, minimal change, IgA nephropathy, and many others. Treatment is mainly directed at the underlying malignancy.[28] Newly discovered antigens such as thrombospondin type-1 domain-containing 7A as well as autoantibodies to neural epidermal growth factor-like 1 and protocadherin 7 have helped in differentiating membranous nephropathy associated with malignancy from the primary form.[29]

Multiple myeloma

The most common kidney involvement in MM is myeloma cast nephropathy (MCN). Casts form as a result of interaction between high concentrations of urinary free light chains (FLC) with uromodulin or Tamm-Horsfall protein. Prompt reduction of FLCs is important to kidney function recovery.[30–32]

Management of MCN mainly involves treating MM and supportive care including IV fluids to maintain a high urine output (above 3 L per day). Hypercalcemia can be managed by IV hydration, bisphosphonates, or receptor activator of nuclear factor (kappa)-B ligand (RANKL) inhibitors.[30]

Lymphoma/leukemia

Renal infiltration is common with leukemias and lymphomas resulting in a wide range of renal dysfunction from asymptomatic to severe needing dialysis. AKI is common in lymphoma and leukemia mainly as pre-renal or ATI. Glomerular disorders associated with leukemia and lymphoma include minimal change disease, focal segmental glomerulosclerosis (FSGS), membranous nephropathy, IgA nephropathy and others. Kidney function may remain normal with these pathologies.[33,34]

Monoclonal gammopathy of renal significance (MGRS) Monoclonal proteins are nephrotoxic by nature which is well-established in MM. MGRS is a term used when kidney damage is a result of these proteins produced by smaller amounts of clones without meeting standard criteria for malignancies such as MM or lymphoma. Treatment is based on targeting the underlying clone.[30]

ELECTROLYTE DISORDERS IN THE CANCER PATIENTS

Abnormalities in serum electrolytes commonly occur in cancer patients, particularly hyponatremia, hypomagnesemia, hypokalemia, and hypercalcemia, due to malignancy or its treatment.

Hyponatremia

Hyponatremia is common in cancer patients. Incidence rates are variable depending on the type of cancer or care setting. In the HYPNOSIS study, 27% of inpatient oncology admissions had hyponatremia.[35] Although most were characterized as mild–moderate, 4.3% had severe hyponatremia (Na<125 mEq/L). In another study of patients facing end-of-life, 8% had moderate hyponatremia whereas 4.3% had severe hyponatremia.[36] Importantly, hyponatremia is associated with increased mortality compared with normonatremic controls.[35]

Management of hyponatremia in cancer patients follows the same principles as the general population. **Fig. 1** illustrates a practical, cancer-specific approach to hyponatremia, beginning with confirming hypotonicity. Clinical status, urine osmolarity, and urine sodium determine whether water excess in hyponatremia reflects elevated anti-diuretic hormone (ADH) and whether high ADH is physiologically inappropriate (syndrome of inappropriate ADH or syndrome of inappropriate anti-diuresis [SIADH]) or not (decreased effective circulating volume). Treatment of hyponatremia depends on etiology, chronicity, severity, and clinical setting. Chronic hyponatremia should not be corrected >6 to 8 mEq over 24 hours.[37] Fluid restriction is necessary but insufficient if the sum of urine sodium and urine potassium > serum sodium. Additional interventions include hypertonic saline for patients with neurologic symptoms. Loop diuretics, salt tablets, urea, and ADH receptor antagonists may all be used in acute and chronic management of hyponatremia secondary to SIADH. Recent reviews and guidelines discuss this in detail.[37,38]

Hypomagnesemia

Magnesium (Mg) is an abundant intracellular cation important to glucose metabolism, skeletal and cardiac myocyte function, and blood pressure regulation.[39] Hypomagnesemia (Mg < 1.8 mg/dL) is asymptomatic till severe deficiency (<1.2 mg/dL) causes muscle cramps, constipation, or other electrolyte disorders including hypokalemia or hypocalcemia.[39] Hypomagnesemia may result from reduced intake, blunted gastrointestinal absorption (proton pump inhibitors), or increased gastrointestinal losses (diarrhea). In cancer patients, anti-neoplastic drugs such as cetuximab, cisplatin, and anti-human epidermal growth factor receptor-2 (HER2) agents inhibit active

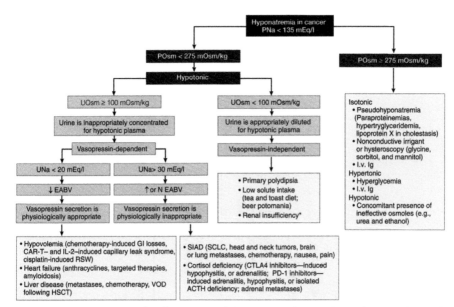

Fig. 1. A diagnostic approach to hyponatremia in cancer patients. ACTH, adrenocorticotropin hormone; CAR-T, chimeric antigen receptor T-cell; CTLA4, cytotoxic T-lymphocyte-associated 4; EABV, effective arterial blood volume; HSCT, hematopoietic stem cell transplant; IL-2, interleukin 2; PD-1, programmed cell death-1; PNa, plasma sodium; POsm, plasma osmolarity; RSW, renal salt wasting; SCLC, small cell lung cancer; SIAD, syndrome of inappropriate anti-diuresis, traditionally referred to as SIADH; TURP, transurethral resection of the prostate; Una, urine sodium; UOsm, urine osmolarity; VOD, veno-occlusive disease. *, urine osmolality in patients with renal insufficiency may be less than plasma osmolality, but is usually not maximally dilute. (*From* Biruh T. Workeneh, Kenar D. Jhaveri, Helbert Rondon-Berrios, Hyponatremia in the cancer patient, Kidney International, Volume 98, Issue 4, 2020, Pages 870-882, ISSN 0085-2538, https://doi.org/10.1016/j.kint.2020.05.015. [https://www.sciencedirect.com/science/article/pii/S0085253820305597].)

reabsorption of Mg at the distal nephron and cause renal Mg wasting.[40] Calcineurin inhibitors for prophylaxis against graft-versus-host disease in allogeneic stem cell transplants similarly induce Mg wasting.[40] Fractional excretion of Mg >2% in patients with normal GFR and hypomagnesemia supports renal wasting. Dose titration of supplements such as Mg sulfate is limited by diarrheal side effects. Mg lactate or Mg chloride preparations may be better tolerated in our anecdotal experience. In severe cases, concurrent use of amiloride may increase Mg reabsorption in the collecting duct.[41]

Hypercalcemia

Calcium homeostasis is a balance between bone formation (osteoblastic) and bone breakdown (osteoclastic). Hypercalcemia, which has been reported to affect 30% of patients with malignancy and portends poor prognosis, occurs when increased osteoclastic activity is not met with sufficient compensatory responses (ie, increased renal calcium excretion).[42] Central to increased osteoclastic activity is interaction between RANK on osteoclasts (or precursor) and RANKL on osteoblasts.[43] This may happen via humoral hypercalcemia of malignancy (HHM) when tumors, usually squamous cell, secrete parathyroid-related protein (PTHrP). Some tumors may secrete parathyroid hormone (PTH) while other cancers upregulate 1-alpha-hydroxylase enzymatic activity to increase 25-hydroxyvitamin D conversion to 1,25-dihydroxyvitamin D

Table 2
Low potassium levels in cancer patients have multiple causes, both cancer-specific and cancer-independent

			Etiology of Low Potassium Levels			
	Decreased Intake	Pseudo-Hypokalemia	Cellular Translocation	Gastrointestinal Losses	Renal Losses
Specific to Cancer	• Cancer cachexia • Dysphagia from obstructing tumor	• Leukocytosis from CLL, AML, etc.	• AML blast crisis	• VIPoma, secretory villous adenoma	• AML with renin production • ACTH-producing tumors
Not-specific to Cancer	• Chemotherapy-induced dysgeusia, nausea • Chemotherapy-associated mucositis	• Leukocytosis from non-malignant causes	• GM-CSF • Vitamin B12	• Radiation or chemotherapy-induced vomiting/diarrhea	• Chemo-induced Fanconi syndrome • Lysozymuria

Abbreviations: ACTH, adrenocorticotropin hormone; AML, acute myelogenous leukemia; CLL, chronic lymphocytic leukemia; GM-CSF, granulocyte-macrophage colony stimulating factor; VIP, vasoactive intestinal peptide.

that increases intestinal calcium absorption.[43] PTH and PTHrP increase RANK-RANKL signaling and counter urinary calcium excretion.[43] Primary or metastatic bone tumors secrete cytokines that directly upregulate RANKL for lytic calcium release from bone.[43]

Hypercalcemia may be asymptomatic if mild but levels >13 mg/dL may present with mental status change, constipation, and nausea/vomiting. Treatment focuses on volume expansion with saline to increase calciuresis. Loop diuretics were once suggested for increased distal nephron sodium delivery to increase urine calcium excretion, but this has been proven to be ineffective or counterproductive as a primary therapy.[44] Calcitonin stimulates calciuresis and inhibits osteoclasts but decreases in calcium are short-lived due to tachyphylaxis.[42,43] Bisphosphonates inhibit osteoclasts but are associated with FSGS (pamidronate)[45] and ATI (zoledronic acid).[46] RANKL inhibitors including denosumab may be the better option in patients with eGFR <60.

Hypokalemia/Hyperkalemia

Hyperkalemia is less common than hypokalemia in the malignancy setting, usually occurring in the context of TLS or AKI of any cause. Pseudohyperkalemia may be noted when fragile leukemic cells lyse during the centrifugation process of measuring serum potassium and is ruled out if a subsequent plasma sample reveals normokalemia.[47]

Pseudohypokalemia may also be reported with severe leukocytosis when dividing cells in blood samples stored at room temperature uptake serum potassium.[48] Rapid fractionation of serum or plasma from the cellular component or refrigeration of the blood sample avoids pseudohypokalemia. Confirmed hypokalemia in the cancer patient may be directly related to the particular malignancy or only indirectly related to it (**Table 2**). For example, acute myeloid leukemia (AML) may specifically release lysozyme to induce proximal tubular injury and potassium loss or treatment of AML may result in diarrhea that leads to potassium loss. Treatment of hypokalemia depends on severity and etiology. In general, hypomagnesemia should be corrected and repletion of potassium stores in cancer patients follows the same guidelines as non-cancer patients.[49]

SUMMARY

Patients facing cancer have a high likelihood of experiencing AKI, CKD, proteinuria, and/or electrolyte disorders during their post-diagnosis clinical course. These manifestations of kidney disease require prompt evaluation by nephrologists experienced in the care of such patients. Major hospitals now have specialized Onco-Nephrology clinics and we recommend that patients with kidney disease, particularly those with AKI, CKD III, or higher, high-grade (>1.5 g) proteinuria, uncontrolled hypertension, and refractory electrolyte derangements be referred to such clinics.

CLINICS CARE POINTS

- Kidney disease in cancer patients may result in acute kidney injury, chronic kidney disease, proteinuria and/or electrolyte disorders.
- Depending on the malignancy and the cancer, kidney disease in cancer patients may be due to specific effects of the cancer or cancer-directed treatments.
- Given the complexity of care of kidney disease in cancer patients, referral to nephrology is essential and when available, referral to onco-nephrology is advisable.

DISCLOSURES

A.C. Shirali-consultant for OnViv.

REFERENCES

1. Christiansen CF, Johansen MB, Langeberg WJ, et al. Incidence of acute kidney injury in cancer patients: a Danish population-based cohort study. Eur J Intern Med 2011;22(4):399–406.
2. Kitchlu Abhijat, McArthur Eric, Amir Eitan, et al. Acute Kidney Injury in Patients Receiving Systemic Treatment for Cancer: A Population-Based Cohort Study. JNCI 2019;111(7):727–36.
3. Launay-Vacher V, Oudard S, Janus N, et al. Renal Insufficiency and Cancer Medications (IRMA) Study Group. Prevalence of Renal Insufficiency in cancer patients and implications for anticancer drug management: the renal insufficiency and anticancer medications (IRMA) study. Cancer 2007;110(6):1376–84.
4. Ciorcan M, Chisavu L, Mihaescu A, et al. Chronic kidney disease in cancer patients, the analysis of a large oncology database from Eastern Europe. PLoS One 2022;17(6):e0265930.
5. Salahudeen AK, Doshi SM, Pawar T, et al. Incidence rate, clinical correlates, and outcomes of AKI in patients admitted to a comprehensive cancer center. Clin J Am Soc Nephrol 2013;8(3):347–54.
6. Herget-Rosenthal S, Marggraf G, Hüsing J, et al. Early detection of acute renal failure by serum cystatin C. Kidney Int 2004;66(3):1115–22.
7. Rosner MH, Jhaveri KD, McMahon BA, et al. Onconephrology: The intersections between the kidney and cancer. CA Cancer J Clin 2021;71(1):47–77.
8. Smith ER, Cai MM, McMahon LP, et al. The value of simultaneous measurements of urinary albumin and total protein in proteinuric patients. Nephrol Dial Transplant 2012;27(4):1534–41.
9. Bonilla M, et al. Onconephrology 2022: an Update. Kidney360 2022. https://doi.org/10.34067/KID.0001582022.
10. García-Carro C, Draibe J, Soler MJ. Onconephrology: Update in Anticancer drug-related nephrotoxicity. Nephron 2022.
11. Rosner MH, Perazella MA. Acute kidney injury in the patient with cancer. Kidney Res Clin Pract 2019;38(3):295–308.
12. Gupta S, Portales-Castillo I, Daher A, et al. Conventional Chemotherapy Nephrotoxicity. Adv Chron Kidney Dis 2021;28(5):402.e1–414.e1.
13. Dobyan DC, Levi J, Jacobs C, et al. Mechanism of cis-platinum nephrotoxicity: II. Morphologic observations. J Pharmacol Exp Ther 1980 Jun;213(3):551–6.
14. Stewart DJ, Dulberg CS, Mikhael NZ, et al. Association of cisplatin nephrotoxicity with patient characteristics and cisplatin administration methods. Cancer Chemother Pharmacol 1997;40:293–308.
15. Arany I, Safirstein RL. Cisplatin nephrotoxicity. Semin Nephrol 2003;23(5):460–4.
16. Barreto JN, Kashani KB, Mara KC, et al. A Prospective Evaluation of Novel Renal Biomarkers in Patients With Lymphoma Receiving High-Dose Methotrexate. Kidney Int Rep 2022;7(7):1690–3.
17. Truong H, Leung N. Fixed-Dose Glucarpidase for Toxic Methotrexate Levels and Acute Kidney Injury in Adult Lymphoma Patients: Case Series. Clin Lymphoma, Myeloma & Leukemia 2021;21(6):e497–502.
18. Ensergueix G, Pallet N, Joly D, et al. Ifosfamide nephrotoxicity in adult patients. Clin Kidney J 2019;13(4):660–5.

19. Ruf R, Yarandi N, Ortiz-Melo DI, et al. Onco-hypertension: Overview of hypertension with anti-cancer agents. J Onco-Nephrol 2021;5(1):57–69.

20. Rashidi A, Wanchoo R, Izzedine H. How I manage hypertension and proteinuria associated with VEGF inhibitor. Clinical Journal of the American Society of Nephrology 2022. CJN.05610522.

21. Sy-Go JPT, Yarandi N, Schwartz GL, et al. Ribociclib-Induced Pseudo-Acute Kidney Injury. J Onco-Nephrol 2022;6(1–2):64–9.

22. Gupta S, Caza T, Herrmann SM, et al. Clinicopathologic Features of Acute Kidney Injury Associated With CDK4/6 Inhibitors. Kidney Int Rep 2022;7(3):618–23.

23. Herrmann SM, Perazella MA. Immune Checkpoint Inhibitors and Immune-Related Adverse Renal Events. Kidney International Reports 2020;5(8):1139–48.

24. Gupta S, Short SAP, Sise ME, et al. Acute kidney injury in patients treated with immune checkpoint inhibitors. J Immunother Cancer 2021;9(10):e003467.

25. Farooqui N, Sy-Go JPT, Miao J, et al. Incidence and Risk Factors for Acute Kidney Injury After Chimeric Antigen Receptor T-Cell Therapy. Mayo Clin Proc 2022; 97(7):1294–304.

26. Howard SC, Jones DP, Pui C-H. The Tumor Lysis Syndrome. N Engl J Med 2011; 364(19):1844–54.

27. Arnaud M, Loiselle M, Vaganay C, et al. Tumor Lysis Syndrome and AKI: Beyond Crystal Mechanisms. J Am Soc Nephrol 2022;33(6):1154–71.

28. Jeyabalan A, Trivedi M. Paraneoplastic Glomerular Diseases. Adv Chron Kidney Dis 2022;29(2):116–26.e1.

29. Ronco P, Beck L, Debiec H, et al. Membranous nephropathy. Nat Rev Dis Prim 2021;7(1):69.

30. Bridoux F, Cockwell P, Glezerman I, et al. Kidney injury and disease in patients with haematological malignancies. Nat Rev Nephrol 2021;17:386.

31. Yadav P, Sathick IJ, Leung N, et al. Serum free light chain level at diagnosis in myeloma cast nephropathy—a multicentre study. Blood Cancer J 2020;10(3):28.

32. Rajkumar SV, Dimopoulos MA, Palumbo A, et al. International Myeloma Working Group updated criteria for the diagnosis of multiple myeloma. Lancet Oncol 2014;15(12):e538–48.

33. Luciano RL, Brewster UC. Kidney Involvement in Leukemia and Lymphoma. Adv Chron Kidney Dis 2014;21(1):27–35.

34. Wanchoo R, Jhaveri KD, Deray G, et al. Renal effects of BRAF inhibitors: a systematic review by the Cancer and the Kidney International Network. Clin Kidney J 2016;9(2):245–51.

35. Fucà G, Mariani L, Lo Vullo S, et al. Weighing the prognostic role of hyponatremia in hospitalized patients with metastatic solid tumors: the HYPNOSIS study. Sci Rep 2019;9(12993).

36. Ferraz Gonçalves J, Brandão M, Arede A, et al. Hyponatremia in Cancer Patients Hospitalized in a Palliative Care Department: A Cross-Sectional Analysis. Acta Med Port 2022;35(2):105–10.

37. Verbalis JG, Goldsmith SR, Greenberg A, et al. Diagnosis, evaluation, and treatment of hyponatremia: expert panel recommendations. Am J Med 2013;126(10 Suppl 1):S1–42.

38. Workeneh BT, Jhaveri KD, Rondon-Berrios H. Hyponatremia in the cancer patient. Kidney Int 2020;98(4):870–82.

39. Gröber U, Schmidt J, Kisters K. Magnesium in Prevention and Therapy. Nutrients 2015;7(9):8199–226.

40. Workeneh BT, Uppal NN, Jhaveri KD, et al. Hypomagnesemia in the Cancer Patient. Kidney360 2020;2(1):154–66.

41. Martin KJ, González EA, Slatopolsky E. Clinical consequences and management of hypomagnesemia. J Am Soc Nephrol 2009;20(11):2291–5.
42. Stewart AF. Clinical practice. Hypercalcemia associated with cancer. N Engl J Med 2005;352(4):373–9.
43. Guise TA, Wysolmerski JJ. Cancer-Associated Hypercalcemia. N Engl J Med 2022;386(15):1443–51.
44. LeGrand SB, Leskuski D, Zama I. Narrative review: furosemide for hypercalcemia: an unproven yet common practice. Ann Intern Med 2008;149:259–63.
45. Markowitz GS, Appel GB, Fine PL, et al. Collapsing focal segmental glomerulosclerosis following treatment with high-dose pamidronate. J Am Soc Nephrol 2001;12(6):1164–72.
46. Markowitz GS, Fine PL, Stack JI, et al. Toxic acute tubular necrosis following treatment with zoledronate (Zometa). Kidney Int 2003;64(1):281–9.
47. Colussi G, Cipriani D. Pseudohyperkalemia in extreme leukocytosis. Am J Nephrol 1995;15:450–2.
48. Naparstek Y, Gutman A. Case report: spurious hypokalemia in myeloproliferative disorders. Am J Med Sci 1984;288:175–7.
49. Unwin RJ, Luft FC, Shirley DG. Pathophysiology and management of hypokalemia: a clinical perspective. Nat Rev Nephrol 2011;7(2):75–84.

Updates in Cardiorenal Syndrome

Wendy McCallum, MD, MS[a],*, Jeffrey M. Testani, MD, MTR[b]

KEYWORDS

- Cardiorenal syndrome • Acute decompensated heart failure • Venous congestion
- Neurohormonal activation

KEY POINTS

- Cardiorenal syndrome is an umbrella term that recognizes the interorgan relationship between the kidneys and the heart and how injury to one organ often leads to injury in the other
- The pathophysiology of cardiorenal syndrome is complex and heterogenous, but includes hemodynamic changes and neurohormonal upregulation among other etiologies
- Management for ADHF remains focused on decongestion with diuretics as well as neurohormonal modulation as a way to overcome the intense sodium and fluid avidity of the CRS.

INTRODUCTION

Among patients with heart failure, there is a high prevalence of chronic kidney disease (CKD), with both disorders sharing significant common risk factors. Dysfunction in both the heart and kidney has been collectively grouped under the term cardiorenal syndrome (CRS). There have been attempts to define CRS by subtypes, according to which organ—the heart versus the kidney—is believed to be the culprit organ triggering dysfunction in the other. However, in most clinical settings, it is challenging to delineate because the pathophysiology is closely intertwined and pathways remain poorly understood. For the purposes of this review in CRS, we will primarily focus on 2 patient populations—patients with chronic heart failure in the ambulatory setting and patients admitted to the hospital for acute decompensated heart failure (ADHF)—and review the kidney complications that can arise in these 2 clinical scenarios and updates in pharmacologic treatment options.

[a] Division of Nephrology, Tufts Medical Center, 800 Washington Street, Box 391, Boston, MA 02111, USA; [b] Division of Cardiovascular Medicine, Yale School of Medicine, PO Box 208017, New Haven, CT 06520, USA
* Corresponding author. 800 Washington Street, Box 391, Boston, MA 02111, USA
E-mail address: wmccallum@tuftsmedicalcenter.org

Med Clin N Am 107 (2023) 763–780
https://doi.org/10.1016/j.mcna.2023.03.011
0025-7125/23/© 2023 Elsevier Inc. All rights reserved.
medical.theclinics.com

EPIDEMIOLOGY AND PROGNOSIS

The prevalence of heart failure is estimated around 64.3 million adults worldwide.[1] Among patients with heart failure, the prevalence of CKD, as defined by an estimated glomerular filtration rate (eGFR) of <60 mL/min/1.73 m^2, is upwards of 50%.[2] The presence of CKD is one of the most powerful risk factors for mortality and cardiovascular events among patients with heart failure.[3] Multiple observational studies and post-hoc analyses have shown a graded association between eGFR and risk for mortality, with risks highest among those with the lowest eGFR.[4]

Fluctuations in eGFR are also very commonly encountered among patients with heart failure. In many other patient populations, an acute decline in eGFR is often interpreted as a clinical cue for either decline in clinical status or a sign of kidney injury in reaction to drugs or other substances. However, given the frequent fluid shifts and medication-associated hemodynamic declines in eGFR that can be observed with many classes of cardioprotective medications (such as with renin-angiotensin-aldosterone system [RAAS] inhibitors), interpreting acute eGFR declines among patients with heart failure can be challenging. For example, among patients admitted for ADHF, the prevalence of acute eGFR declines has been shown to be around 20% to 30%.[5] Unlike baseline reduced eGFR, these acute eGFR changes are not as consistently associated with adverse clinical outcomes. Particularly if the acute eGFR decline is sustained after an intervention that is otherwise protective in heart failure—whether it is diuresis for ADHF or initiation of a RAAS inhibitor—the cardiovascular benefits of the intervention outweigh any risk associated with the eGFR decline. Post-hoc analysis of the ESCAPE trial,[6] which randomized patients admitted for ADHF to treatment guided by a pulmonary artery catheter versus without, showed that acute declines in eGFR that occurred together with simultaneous evidence of hemoconcentration (as a proxy of decongestion), were not associated with greater risks of mortality and rehospitalization for ADHF.[7] In contrast, if an acute decline in eGFR is sustained outside of interventions such as diuresis or initiation of RAAS inhibitor—such as ongoing congestion in the hospital—the acute eGFR decline likely signals a decline in clinical status and thereby associated with adverse outcomes such as higher risk of mortality and re-hospitalization for heart failure. A number of studies drawn from different ADHF trials have shown consistent findings, reiterating the importance of context for interpreting acute eGFR declines among patients with heart failure.[8,9]

PATHOPHYSIOLOGY AND COMPLICATIONS

The mechanisms underlying the pathophysiology of the CRS are not well understood, but most likely involve multiple bi-directional pathways centering on arterial underfilling, venous congestion, and neurohormonal activation.

Arterial Underfilling

While historically it had been believed that low cardiac output was the primary driver of low GFR in the CRS, there have since been multiple observational studies showing no direct association between low cardiac output and either reduced baseline eGFR or acute declines in eGFR.[10,11] There have also been several trials of therapeutic agents that increase cardiac output, without clear evidence of any connection between increasing the cardiac output and an increase in eGFR. In the OPTIME-CHF trial, in which 951 patients with ADHF were randomized to treatment with 48-h of milrinone versus placebo, the use of milrinone as a positive inotropic agent did not show any associated increases in eGFR.[12,13] Some of the inotropic effects could have been off-set by the vasodilating effects of milrinone, with about 10% having sustained hypotension (systolic blood pressure<80 mm Hg) compared to 3% in the placebo arm. However, the GALACTIC trial, a large randomized control trial of the selective cardiac myosin activator, omecamtiv mecarbil, also failed to show any increases in eGFR in the treatment arm.[14] Of the 4120 patients randomized to the omecamtiv mecarbil group, a drug that directly augments cardiac sarcomere function and known to improve stroke volume, there was no change in serum creatinine at 48 weeks and no difference between the treatment arm and placebo arm (creatinine change of 0.06 ± 0.39 mg/dL in the treatment arm vs 0.05 ± 0.38 mg/dL in the placebo arm). In other words, low cardiac output in ADHF might be triggering a cascade of maladaptive responses, but overall does not seem to be the main driver of declines in eGFR on a population level. On the other hand, there are certain scenarios such as cardiogenic shock, an extreme case of low cardiac output and of low organ perfusion that leads to organ ischemia, including the kidney, where this relationship is likely highly relevant.

Venous Congestion

There has been literature suggesting that in cross-sectional studies, venous congestion as measured by elevated central venous pressures (CVP), can be associated with low baseline kidney function.[11,15] However, this has been an inconsistent finding and on average across studies rarely is CVP anything more than weakly associated with renal function. The challenge remains even when evaluating the weak association, more severe venous congestion in ADHF is often associated with more severe heart failure, making it very difficult to isolate whether the congestion itself is associated with lower kidney function, or whether patients with more advanced and severe heart failure have more diuretic resistance and worse kidney function by virtue of having more advanced cardiac disease. Furthermore, in terms of longitudinal changes in eGFR, neither higher CVP nor changes in CVP have been associated with either declines or increases in eGFR over the course of hospitalization for ADHF.[11,16,17] Overall, however, congestion is consistently associated with poor survival and re-hospitalization for ADHF, making decongestion and maintaining euvolemia an important priority from a cardiovascular perspective, regardless of whether the eGFR decreases or increases. While decongestion has not been associated with improvements in eGFR, one observational study has at least shown no evidence of longer term kidney function declines among those with more rapid in-hospital decongestion.[18] While the congestion itself may not be the primary factor driving declines in kidney function, such patients with greater excess venous congestion and diminished ability to respond to diuretics will be at much higher risk of mortality and morbidity, including declines in kidney function.

Neurohormonal Activity, Sodium, and Water Avidity

The hallmark of the CRS is intense sodium and water avidity, leading to fluid retention and diminished urinary response to diuretics. There are a number of neurohormonal pathways that drive kidney sodium and water avidity, including components of the RAAS such as angiotensin II, aldosterone, as well as the sympathetic nervous system and vasopressin. Arterial underfilling in heart failure will stimulate baroreceptors to trigger RAAS stimulation; on the other hand, some animal studies of renal vein ligation have also shown an increase in RAAS activity and urine sodium avidity with venous renal congestion as well.[19] Another important trigger for RAAS is low tubular fluid chloride delivery sensed by the macula densa. Observational studies have shown that renin levels are higher among patients with hypochloremia, with plasma renin levels correlated negatively with serum chloride values even after adjustment for baseline kidney function.[20]

The other important neurohormonal axis is the natriuretic peptide system. Volume overload and myocardial stretch have been shown to release natriuretic peptides, which counteract many of the sodium avidity triggers described above. Natriuretic peptide receptors in the kidney will stimulate sodium excretion and increase GFR. Administration of recombinant natriuretic peptides such as nesiritide showed improvements in cardiac and renal hemodynamics in some short-term studies[21,22]; however, in larger trials among patients with ADHF, there were no improvements in either urine output, eGFR, or cardiovascular outcomes.[23,24]

DIAGNOSTIC STRATEGIES
Evaluations of Kidney Function: Blood Biomarkers

There are many nuances to how to evaluate kidney function among patients with heart failure. There are no current biomarkers that are able to capture all the various functions that the kidney accomplishes—in other words, not just glomerular filtration, but also tubular electrolyte and water handling and endocrine functions. Serum creatinine is the most widely available biomarker and remains the backbone of GFR estimating equations including the updated CKD-EPI 2021 formula.[25] However, it is important to acknowledge the limitations of creatinine, particularly factors that can impact the value of serum creatinine outside of GFR. Creatinine is a by-product of muscle metabolism, and therefore patients with low muscle mass can have low values of serum creatinine that can lead to over-estimates of their kidney function. Particularly for patients with heart failure, among whom there is a high prevalence of sarcopenia and muscle loss, an eGFR based on creatinine can be an overestimate of the measured GFR. Several medications, such as trimethoprim or cimetidine, can block the tubular secretion of creatinine and conversely lead to an underestimate of the GFR. These nuances to interpretation can become important when patients are being considered candidates for certain medication classes, antibiotic dosing, and candidacy for advanced therapies.

Another biomarker that has become more widely available for clinical use is cystatin C, a low molecular weight protein ubiquitously expressed throughout all nucleated cells. For the general population, it has been recommended to incorporate both creatinine and cystatin C into the CKD-EPI 2021 formula for better accuracy.[26] While cystatin C may be less affected by muscle mass relative to creatinine, it can be affected by other factors such as thyroid disease, steroid use, smoking, and inflammation.[27] The nuances of interpretation of cystatin C among patients with heart failure is still an area that needs greater evaluation.

In terms of monitoring changes in kidney function, a rise in serum creatinine is a relatively delayed finding in intrinsic kidney injury. Furthermore, a rise in creatinine can also occur when there are hemodynamic changes to GFR, without injury. Among patients with heart failure, who are prone to hemodynamic fluid shifts, but also at risk for ischemic tubular injury, an acute rise in serum creatinine becomes a challenging finding to interpret. In a post-hoc analysis of the ROSE-AHF study, levels of tubular injury biomarkers—including N-acetyl-β-D-glucosaminidase (NAG), kidney injury molecule-1 (KIM-1) and neutrophil gelatinase-associated lipocalin (NGAL)—did not change with protocol-driven diuresis (median urine output of 8.4 L over 72-h), whereas the eGFR decreased by $\geq$ 20% in 21% of patients.[28] There was also no association between eGFR decline and increase in the tubular injury biomarkers, suggesting that these were not signs of intrinsic kidney injury. However, other studies have observed elevation in levels of NGAL with diuresis that were not associated with mortality events or development of kidney failure.[29] With the inconsistency of results, none of the tubular injury biomarkers are being recommended for routine clinical use at this time.

Evaluations of Kidney Function: Urinary Tests

Examination of the urine can be a helpful piece of clinical data in the evaluation of the CRS. A urinalysis (and if possible, examination of the urine sediment) is classically believed to be bland (ie, no red blood cells or white blood cells or casts) if the decline in kidney function is in the setting of CRS. On the other hand, any other findings on urinalysis may prompt further investigation and reveal a number of potential etiologies of intrinsic kidney disease such as diabetic nephropathy, interstitial nephritis, acute tubular necrosis, or vasculitis. However, it should be pointed out that since there is no gold standard diagnostic test for CRS, it is challenging to know if an active sediment is in fact never seen in CRS. Particularly among patients with both heart failure and CKD with proteinuria, it would be important not to miss diagnoses such as amyloidosis or Fabry disease, which would lead to a significant change in management. Quantification of proteinuria and albuminuria with the use of spot samples or 24-h urine collection is also helpful. Among patients with ADHF, one study repeated spot urine albumin:creatinine ratios daily over the first 7-days of hospitalization to assess whether the degree of albuminuria changes with decongestion.[30] It showed that the prevalence of albuminuria diminished over time with diuresis; however, an important caveat is that the quantification using spot samples can vary substantially depending on the degree of urinary creatinine excretion measured on each spot sample, which may or may not change during ADHF therapy. Assessment of whether albuminuria changes with decongestion, when measured using 24-h urine collections, would be interesting.

Evaluation of urine electrolytes, in particular urinary sodium, has also become incorporated as a way to evaluate diuretic response among patients admitted for ADHF. A low spot urine sodium obtained ~2 hours after dosing of diuretics can be a good predictor of poor diuretic response and can help guide diuretic dose escalation.[31]

Evaluations of Kidney Function: Imaging Modalities

Imaging of the kidneys can provide some helpful information as well. At least among patients with general CKD, ultrasound findings of echogenicity correlated best with histopathologic findings of chronicity and scarring.[32] Presumably, this correlation could be extrapolated to patients with heart failure as well but has not been formally evaluated. Point-of-care ultrasound, which has been increasingly incorporated into certain clinical settings including the emergency department and intensive care unit, has been investigated as a noninvasive modality to assess venous congestion and aid decision-making regarding diuresis. Patterns of blood flow in the inferior vena cava, hepatic vein, portal vein, and intrarenal veins have been identified as evidence of venous congestion that correlates with elevated central venous pressures.[33] There has also been some interest in using patterns of intrarenal venous blood flow as a prognostic tool,[34] but whether it adds more information on top of other clinical markers of venous congestion is still unknown.

MANAGEMENT—CHRONIC HEART FAILURE

For the majority of patients with both heart failure and CKD, with the bi-directional crosstalk from both organs, therapeutic management can focus on therapies that will be cardiac-specific, kidney-specific, or common to both. There have been a number of landmark trials that have changed the landscape of medical management for patients with chronic heart failure and CKD, particularly for heart failure with reduced ejection fraction (HFrEF). For the purposes of this review, we will focus on major classes of agents that have beneficial effects on both the heart and the kidney, including angiotensin receptor/neprilysin inhibitor (ARNI), angiotensin-converting enzyme inhibitor (ACEI), angiotensin II receptor blocker (ARB), mineralocorticoid receptor antagonist (MRA) including non-steroidal MRAs, and sodium-glucose contransporter-2 (SGLT2) inhibitors.

Angiotensin-Converting Enzyme Inhibitors, Angiotensin II Receptor Blockers

Activation of the RAAS hormonal pathway is a compensatory mechanism after cardiac injury, as well as in the setting of perceived arterial underfilling. In terms of the kidney, RAAS will lead to preferential vasoconstriction of the efferent arteriole, increasing intraglomerular pressure. Angiotensin II and aldosterone are also powerful stimulants for sodium reabsorption along multiple points of the renal tubules. Blockade of the RAAS hormonal pathway remains a cornerstone in the management of HFrEF. Multiple landmark trials have shown mortality and cardiovascular benefit in HFrEF (**Table 1**), and blockade using ACEI or ARB also plays a key central role in the management of proteinuric CKD. Because of the many shared comorbidities between CKD and HFpEF—namely diabetes and hypertension—the majority of patients with HFpEF will also meet indications for use of RAAS blockade as demonstrated by a Swedish registry study. Of 16,216 patients enrolled in the Swedish Heart Failure Registry with an EF $\geq$ 40%, 56% were using an ACEI and 20% were using an ARB.[35] In summary, even if trials of RAAS blockade specifically for cardiovascular benefits in HFpEF did not show survival benefit,[36,37] it has been a reasonable recommendation to use these agents to manage other comorbidities such as hypertension or proteinuria.

As alluded to above, an acute decrease in eGFR can be observed after initiating an ACEI or ARB due to the preferential vasodilation of the efferent arteriole leading to a hemodynamic eGFR decline. For example, the SOLVD trials, which randomized patients with HFrEF to treatment with enalapril versus placebo, had collectively about 10% of patients with an acute decline of >20% eGFR decline at 2-weeks. Among the patients with an acute eGFR decline after the initiation of enalapril, the treatment still showed a significant reduction in risk for mortality and hospitalization for ADHF when compared to patients with acute eGFR decline after randomization to placebo.[38,39] Even when compared to patients randomized to placebo without any acute eGFR decline (presuming all the acute eGFR decline can be assumed to be medication-drive), randomization to enalapril still showed clinical benefits.[39]

Angiotensin Receptor/Neprilysin Inhibitor

Natriuretic peptide release is triggered by numerous stimuli, including myocardial stretch from volume overload or other mechanical stressors to the heart. In the kidney, natriuretic peptides counteract many of the actions of RAAS by antagonizing sodium reabsorption and vasoconstriction, resulting in natriuresis. However, infusion of recombinant natriuretic peptides has not shown any benefits such as increase in urinary output or increases in eGFR,[24] nor differences in mortality.[23] Inhibition of neprilysin, a metalloproteinase that degrades natriuretic peptides, has on the other hand been shown to be beneficial for cardiovascular outcomes among patients with HFrEF when used in combination with ARB. The PARADIGM trial randomized 8442 patients with HFrEF to treatment with either sacubitril/valsartan or enalapril, with a decreased risk of cardiovascular death and HF hospitalization observed in the sacubitril/valsartan arm.[40] While randomization to sacubitril/valsartan did not reach statistical significance for benefit in terms of the pre-specified kidney composite endpoint (kidney failure, $\geq$50% eGFR decline, or eGFR decrease by > 30 mL/min/1.73 m^2 to <60 mL/min/1.73 m^2), there was a slower

Table 1
Examples of landmark trials that have influenced pharmacological management of patients with heart failure with reduced ejection fraction

Class of Drug	Trial	n	Intervention	Kidney Exclusion Criteria	Primary Outcome	Kidney Outcome[a]
ARNI	PARADIGM[40]	8442	Sacubitril/valsartan vs enalapril	eGFR <30 mL/min/1.73 m²	HR 0.80 (0.73, 0.87) for composite of CV death or HF hospitalization	eGFR decline by −1.61 mL/min/1.73 m²/year in treatment arm vs −2.04 mL/min/1.73 m²/year in the placebo arm (P < .001)[41] HR 0.86 (0.65, 1.13) for kidney failure, ≥50% eGFR decline, or eGFR decrease by > 30 mL/min/1.73 m² to <60 mL/min/1.73 m²
ACEI	SOLVD- Treatment[69]	2569	Enalapril vs placebo	Cr > 2 mg/dL	RR 0.84 (0.74, 0.95) for all-cause mortality RR 0.74 (0.66, 0.82) for composite of death or HF hospitalization	Initial decline in eGFR in the enalapril arm, without significant difference in longer-term slope thereafter (−0.84 [−1.24, −0.43] vs −1.36 [−1.77, −0.94] mL/min/1.73 m²/yr in the enalapril and placebo arms, respectively)[70]
ACEI	SOLVD-Prevention[71]	4228	Enalapril vs placebo	Cr > 2 mg/dL	RR 0.92 (0.79, 1.08) for all-cause mortality RR 0.64 (0.54, 0.78) for HF hospitalization	Initial decline in eGFR in the enalapril arm, without significant difference in longer-term slope thereafter (−1.27 [−1.56, −0.99] vs −1.37 [−1.65, −1.07] mL/min/1.73 m²/year in the enalapril and placebo arms, respectively)[70]

(continued on next page)

Table 1
(continued)

Class of Drug	Trial	n	Intervention	Kidney Exclusion Criteria	Primary Outcome	Kidney Outcome[a]
MRA	EMPHASIS-HF[72]	2737	Eplerenone vs placebo	eGFR <30 mL/min/1.73 m²	HR 0.63 (0.54, 0.74) for composite of CV death or HF hospitalization	Initial faster rate of decline in eGFR in the eplerenone arm (−0.288 mL/min/1.73 m²/year [−0.395, −0.182]) than placebo arm (−0.066 mL/min/1.73 m²/year [−0.174, −0.042]) that was maintained through the trial[73]
MRA	EPHESUS[74]	6632	Eplerenone vs placebo	Cr > 2.5 mg/dL and K > 5 mmol/L	RR 0.85 (0.75, 0.96) for all-cause mortality	Initial decline in eGFR in the eplerenone arm that was maintained through the trial (adjusted mean difference of −1.4 mL/min/1.73 m²)
SGLT2i	DAPA-HF[75]	4744	Dapagliflozin vs placebo	eGFR <30 mL/min/1.73 m²	HR 0.74 (0.65, 0.85) for composite of worsening HF or CV death	eGFR decline by −1.09 mL/min/1.73 m²/year in treatment arm vs −2.85 mL/min/1.73m²/year in the placebo arm (P <.001) HR 0.71 (0.44, 1.16) for renal composite
SGLT2i	EMPEROR-Reduced[76]	3730	Empagliflozin vs placebo	eGFR <20 mL/min/1.73 m²	HR 0.75 (0.65, 0.86) for composite of CV death or HF hospitalization	eGFR decline by −0.55 mL/min/1.73 m²/year in treatment arm vs −2.28 mL/min/1.73m²/year in the placebo arm (P <.001)

Abbreviations: ACEI, angiotensin-converting enzyme inhibitor; ARNI, angiotensin receptor-neprilysin inhibitor; Cr, creatinine; CV, cardiovascular; eGFR, estimated glomerular filtration rate; HF, heart failure; K, potassium; MRA, mineralocorticoid receptor antagonist; SGLT2i, sodium/glucose cotransporter-2 inhibitor.
[a] Some kidney endpoints were prespecified endpoints from the original trial, and some were from post-hoc analyses; unless separate citation is included, the endpoint was from the original trial.

rate of decrease in eGFR in the sacubitril/valsartan arm. Over the course of follow-up, the eGFR decreased by −1.61 mL/min/1.73 m²/year (95% CI -1.77 to −1.44 mL/min/1.73 m²/year) among those randomized to sacubitril/valsartan compared to −2.04 mL/min/1.73 m²/year (95% CI -2.21 to −1.88 mL/min/1.73 m²/year; P < .001) among those randomized to placebo[41] (see **Table 1**). Guidelines have incorporated the use of ARNI as first-line recommendation for the management of HFrEF, as long as tolerated from a blood pressure perspective.[42]

In contrast, the PARAGON study, which randomized 4822 patients with HFpEF to treatment with sacubitril/valsartan vs valsartan, only showed a trend toward benefit against cardiovascular outcomes.[43] However, randomization to the sacubitril/valsartan arm showed a 50% decreased risk of a kidney composite outcome of kidney-related death, development of kidney failure or >50% decline in eGFR (HR = 0.50, 95% CI 0.33, 0.77).[44] Furthermore, in a recent analysis of the pooled PARAGON and PARADIGM trials examining this set of composite renal outcomes (slightly modified from the pre-specified outcomes), randomization to sacubitril/valsartan was also associated with decreased risk of the composite outcome defined as ≥50% eGFR decline or development of kidney failure or death due to renal causes (HR = 0.56, 95% CI 0.42, 0.75).[45]

Mineralocorticoid Receptor Antagonists

In the heart, aldosterone has been shown to accelerate pro-fibrotic pathways which lead to hypertrophy, fibrosis, and adverse remodeling. Similarly, in the kidney, aldosterone has been associated with fibrosis with increased tissue production of transforming growth factor beta and fibronectin.[46] Agents such as spironolactone and eplerenone competitively block mineralicorticoid receptors, inhibiting the action of aldosterone. Trials among patients with HFrEF and patients with reduced EF post-myocardial infarction have all shown mortality and cardiovascular benefits with treatment with MRA (see **Table 1**). For patients with HFpEF, the Aldo-DHF trial, which randomized 422 patients with EF ≥ 50% to treatment with spironolactone versus placebo, showed improvement in parameters of diastolic function over the 12-month follow-up.[47] The TOPCAT trial, which included 3445 patients with preserved EF, showed a reduction in the primary outcome of the composite of death, aborted CV death, and HF hospitalization among those randomized to spironolactone over placebo, but it did not meet statistical significance (HR 0.89 [95% CI 0.77, 1.04].[48] However, post-hoc analyses limited to the 1767 patients enrolled in the Americas showed efficacy with spironolactone (HR 0.82 [95% CI 0.69, 0.98]); therefore, guidelines have suggested that there could be potential efficacy for patients with HFpEF.[42]

Given the increased risk of hyperkalemia with treatment with MRAs, as well as fear of hyperkalemia, 2 approaches have been studied: (1) whether continuation of MRAs together with potassium-binding agents is efficacious and safe, and (2) to evaluate non-steroidal MRAs with the belief that they cause less hyperkalemia. The DIAMOND trial included 878 patients with HFrEF with eGFR>30 mL/min/1.73 m² and hyperkalemia (defined as 2 serum potassium values of >5 mmol/L) while taking an ARNI, ACEI, ARB, and/or MRA.[49] Patients were randomized to either patiromer or placebo, while concurrently optimizing RAAS inhibitor therapy including up-titration of the MRA dose up to 50 mg per day. The trial showed that randomization to patiromir was successful in reducing serum potassium levels (between-group difference of −0.10 mmol/L [-0.13, −0.07] in potassium), and in the run-in phase most patients were able to achieve target doses of RAAS inhibitor therapy and MRA. In terms of the theoretical reduction in hyperkalemia risk associated with the non-steroidal MRA finerenone, it has not yet been studied in the heart failure population. The currently enrolling trial

FINEARTS-HF trial (NCT04435626) will be examining finerenone among patients with CKD and HFpEF.

SGLT2 Inhibitors

The sodium-glucose cotransporter-2 reabsorbs glucose and sodium in the proximal tubule of the kidney, and had been initially studied as a target for hypoglycemic agents. Through a thus-far unclear mechanism, blockade of the SGLT2 leads to a wide range of significantly improved clinical outcomes, including overall survival, cardiovascular outcomes, HF hospitalizations, and kidney failure. The use of SGLT2i has become incorporated as first-line therapy in guidelines for both heart failure[42,50] as well as for diabetic kidney disease[51] and other subtypes of proteinuric glomerular disease.[52] With the growing list of patient populations who meet indications for the initiation of SGLT2i—patients with diabetes, diabetic kidney disease with albuminuria, non-diabetic kidney disease with albuminuria (and perhaps soon even without albuminuria), HFrEF, HFpEF and patients with diabetes—there is increased focus on barriers to implementation such as awareness and insurance costs. Particularly among patients with HFpEF, it has become an important class of medications to add to the limited available armamentarium.[53]

MANAGEMENT—ACUTE DECOMPENSATED HEART FAILURE

Hospitalizations for ADHF have accounted for approximately over 1 million hospitalizations in the United States annually,[54] representing a substantial healthcare burden. Most hospitalizations are driven by symptoms of volume overload, and strategies for decongestion remain the mainstay of management for patients admitted with ADHF. Evaluation should include assessment for factors that may have precipitated the ADHF, including acute coronary syndrome, arrhythmias, valvular disease, acute infection, or nonadherence with medication regimens. As for management, many therapeutic agents and strategies for ADHF—including agents to increase cardiac output, antagonize vasoconstriction, and increase urine output and GFR—have been developed but few have shown efficacy in larger trials to improve mortality or rehospitalization for ADHF. Management strategies for ADHF thus remain centered on decongestion and overcoming diuretic resistance, with the caveat that patients that decompensate further into cardiogenic shock would require additional means to restore end-organ perfusion.

Loop Diuretics

Intravenous loop diuretic therapy, which blocks the Na-K-2Cl channel in the kidney's loop of Henle, remains the backbone of decongestive strategies for ADHF. Based on results from the DOSE trial, which showed a trend toward more rapid symptom improvement with high dose over low dose strategies,[55] most clinical practice guidelines recommend initiating an intravenous dose that is 2 times the home daily dose.[42] There was no difference in bolus or continuous dosing. The important goal is to focus on up-titration of dosing within the initial 24-h, using spot urine sodium and/or hourly urine output as data to guide dosing. The European Society of Cardiology has published a position statement recommending a doubling of loop diuretic dose if the spot urine sodium at 2-h post diuretic is < 50 meq/L or the urine output is < 100 mL/h at 6-h post diuretic administration.[31]

Thiazide Diuretics

Thiazide diuretics, which block the Na-Cl cotransporter in the distal convoluted tubule, are important agents to use in combination with loop diuretics. They can be a particularly important class of agents because chronic use of loop diuretics has been shown to lead to distal tubular hypertrophy and increases the abundance of Na-Cl cotransporters.[56] The efficacy of using hydrochlorothiazide combined with a loop diuretic was examined in the Safety and Efficacy of the Combination of Loop with Thiazide-type Diuretics in Patients with Decompensated Heart Failure (CLOROTIC) trial, which randomized 230 patients admitted for ADHF to either thiazide plus loop or loop diuretic alone.[57] The trial showed greater weight loss achieved in the combined arm (−2.3 kg vs −1.5 kg) at 72-h. In contrast to classic teaching, thiazide diuretics — including oral metolazone, oral chlorthalidone, and intravenous chlorothiazide — can be effective at low GFR as well.[58] There can be significant potassium wasting with thiazide diuretics, which would need careful monitoring and repletion.

Mineralocorticoid Receptor Antagonists

Spironolactone and eplerenone act as competitive antagonists of the mineralocorticoid receptor, and are recommended for use in chronic ambulatory management of HFrEF. While they have consistently been shown to reduce risks of mortality and adverse CV outcomes in trials among chronic ambulatory heart failure patient populations, they can play a role as potassium-sparing diuretics for select ADHF patients as well. Even though the ATHENA trial, which randomized 360 patients with ADHF to treatment with high-dose spironolactone (100 mg) versus placebo or low-dose spironolactone (25 mg), did not show a significant difference in urine outcome or weight loss in the hospital, it also did not show any concerns regarding hyperkalemia or eGFR decline.[59] Some of this is related to what was likely inadequate dosing, given the short duration of the trial (4 days) vs the long half-life of the active metabolite of spironolactone, canrenone. Among patients with significant urinary potassium wasting and hypokalemia with diuretic therapy, addition of MRAs may be helpful.

Acetazolamide

Acetazolamide, an inhibitor of carbonic anhydrase, with a site of action primarily in the proximal tubule of the kidney, has generally been incorporated as a diuretic in cases of significant metabolic alkalosis. Blockade of carbonic anhydrase with acetazolamide reduces proton cycling and thereby sodium reabsorption via the sodium/hydrogen exchanger, leading to greater natriuresis. The ADVOR trial, which randomized 519 patients with ADHF to treatment with acetazolamide plus loop diuretic versus placebo plus loop diuretic, showed more rapid decongestion in the treatment arm by 3 days.[60] Notably, augmentation of diuresis/natriuresis was overall modest with 500 mL (95% CI, 200 mL to 800 mL) of additional fluid loss and 98 mmol (95% CI, 56 mmol to 140 mmol) of urine sodium over the 2-day study intervention. There was no significant difference in 3-month mortality or rehospitalization for ADHF, and important to recognize that the trial did not include the use of thiazides or SGLT2 inhibitors.

Vasopressin Antagonists

Tolvaptan, a selective vasopressin V2 antagonist, blocks the insertion of aquaporins into the distal tubule of the kidney and leads to aquaresis. The EVEREST trial, which randomized 4133 patients admitted for ADHF to treatment with tolvaptan versus placebo in addition to standard therapy showed greater weight loss in the tolvaptan arm.[61] However, there was no evidence of benefit in terms of mortality or rehospitalization for ADHF. In a *post-hoc* analysis, there was a cardiovascular benefit among patients with hyponatremia as defined by sodium <130 mmol/L.[62] Addition of tolvaptan could be considered among patients needing additional decongestion and hyponatremia.

Table 2
Examples of trials that have examined pharmacological agents for the management of patients with heart failure with preserved ejection fraction

Class of Drug	Trial	n	Intervention	Kidney Exclusion Criteria	Primary Outcome	Kidney Outcome[a]
ARNI	PARAGON-HF[43]	4822	Sacubitri-valsartan vs valsartan	eGFR <30 mL/min/1.73 m²	RR 0.87 (0.75, 1.01) for composite of CV death or HF hospitalization	HR 0.50 (0.33, 0.77) for composite of death from renal failure, ESKD, or ≥50% eGFR decline[44]
ARB	CHARM-Preserved[36]	3023	Candesartan vs placebo	Cr ≥ 3 mg/dL	HR 0.89 (0.77, 1.03) for composite of CV death or HF hospitalization	Greater decrease in eGFR at 26-mo in the candesartan arm (-9.2 ± 21 mL/min/1.73 m²) vs placebo arm (-3.8 ± 20 mL/min/1.73 m²); $P = .04$
MRA	TOPCAT[7]	3445	Spironolactone vs placebo	eGFR <30 mL/min/1.73 m² or Cr > 2.5 mg/dL	HR 0.89 (0.77, 1.04) for composite of CV death, HF hospitalization, or aborted cardiac arrest	Doubling of serum Cr to a value beyond the upper reference limit was more common in the spironolactone arm than placebo arm (10.2% vs 7.0%, $P < .001$)
SGLT2i	EMPEROR-Preserved[53]	5988	Empagliflozin vs placebo	eGFR <20 mL/min/1.73 m²	HR 0.79 (0.69, 0.90) for composite of CV death or HF hospitalization	eGFR decline by -1.25 mL/min/1.73 m²/year in treatment arm vs -2.62 mL/min/1.73 m²/year in the placebo arm ($P < .001$)

Abbreviations: ACEI, angiotensin-converting enzyme inhibitor; ARNI, angiotensin receptor-neprilysin inhibitor; Cr, creatinine; CV, cardiovascular; eGFR, estimated glomerular filtration rate; ESKD, end stage kidney disease; HF, heart failure; MRA, mineralocorticoid receptor antagonist; SGLT2i, sodium/glucose cotransporter-2 inhibitor.

[a] Some kidney endpoints were prespecified endpoints from the original trial, and some were from post-hoc analyses; unless separate citation is included, the endpoint was from the original trial.

Invasive Methods for Decongestion

If a patient remains volume overloaded despite up-titration of available pharmacologic agents, or there develops the requirement for rapid fluid removal or electrolyte and/or uremic indications for renal replacement therapy (RTT), management could include escalation to invasive means of fluid removal including ultrafiltration or RTT. There have been several trials investigating ultrafiltration versus stepped diuretic therapy suggesting an improvement in rehospitalization; however, this was not observed in all trials.[63–65] Clinical guidance has remained to use pharmacologic therapy until no further options outside of invasive means such as ultrafiltration or RRT for volume removal.

Opportunity to Establish Chronic Heart Failure Therapy

There have been a number of pharmacologic agents incorporated into guideline-directed therapy particularly for chronic ambulatory patients, as outlined in **Table 1** and **Table 2**. However, initiation and maintenance of target dosing of these agents have been shown to fall short in clinical practice.[66] Both patient and clinician apprehension regarding adverse effects—acute eGFR declines, electrolyte abnormalities, blood pressure changes—likely play a large role in the clinical inertia behind slow implementation in the outpatient setting. Studies of various agents have examined the safety and efficacy of initiation of agents such as ARNIs and SGLT2 inhibitors prior to discharge from hospitalization for ADHF and have mostly shown that inpatient initiation is safe.[67,68] Such a strategy of initiation while under close monitoring in the hospital may help address some of the issues of implementation.

SUMMARY

The CRS is a term that refers to a collection of disorders involving both the heart and kidneys, encompassing multi-directional pathways between the 2 organs mediated through low arterial perfusion, venous congestion, and neurohormonal activation. There have been a number of trials of pharmacological agents that have demonstrated improved cardiovascular and kidney outcomes, particularly among chronic ambulatory patients. Management for ADHF remains focused on decongestion and ways to overcome the intense sodium and fluid avidity of the CRS.

CLINICS CARE POINTS

- A low spot urine sodium obtained ~2 hours after dosing of diuretics can be a good predictor of poor diuretic response and can help guide diuretic dose escalation.31

- Patients with cardiorenal syndrome often have diuretic resistance, and will require escalating doses of loop diuretics. When uptitrating the dose of these agents, a doubling of the prior dose should be considered as the next step.

- Neurohormonal modulation in cardiorenal syndrome involves therapy with several classes of therapeutics that have beneficial effects on both the heart and the kidney, these include angiotensin receptor/neprilysin inhibitor (ARNI), angiotensin-converting enzyme inhibitor (ACEI), angiotensin II receptor blocker (ARB), mineralocorticoid receptor antagonist (MRA) including non-steroidal MRAs, and sodium-glucose contransporter-2 (SGLT2) inhibitors.

- Invasive methods for decongestion, such as renal replacement therapy, should be used as a last resort when managing cardiorenal syndrome.

FUNDING

NIH NCATS KL2 (TR002545-04).

REFERENCES

1. GBD 2017 Disease and Injury Incidence and Prevalence Collaborators. Global, regional, and national incidence, prevalence, and years lived with disability for 354 diseases and injuries for 195 countries and territories, 1990-2017: a systematic analysis for the Global Burden of Disease Study 2017. Lancet 2018; 392(10159):1789–858.
2. Damman K, Valente MAE, Voors AA, et al. Renal impairment, worsening renal function, and outcome in patients with heart failure: an updated meta-analysis. Eur Heart J 2014;35(7):455–69.
3. Fonarow GC, Adams KF, Abraham WT, et al. ADHERE Scientific Advisory Committee, Study Group, and Investigators. Risk stratification for in-hospital mortality in acutely decompensated heart failure: classification and regression tree analysis. JAMA 2005;293(5):572–80.
4. Hillege HL, Nitsch D, Pfeffer MA, et al. Renal function as a predictor of outcome in a broad spectrum of patients with heart failure. Circulation 2006;113(5):671–8.
5. Forman DE, Butler J, Wang Y, et al. Incidence, predictors at admission, and impact of worsening renal function among patients hospitalized with heart failure. J Am Coll Cardiol 2004;43(1):61–7. https://doi.org/10.1016/j.jacc.2003.07.031.
6. Binanay C, Califf RM, Hasselblad V, et al. Evaluation study of congestive heart failure and pulmonary artery catheterization effectiveness: the ESCAPE trial. JAMA 2005;294(13):1625–33.
7. Testani JM, Chen J, McCauley BD, et al. Potential effects of aggressive decongestion during the treatment of decompensated heart failure on renal function and survival. Circulation 2010;122(3):265–72.
8. McCallum W, Tighiouart H, Testani JM, et al. Acute Kidney Function Declines in the Context of Decongestion in Acute Decompensated Heart Failure. JACC Heart Fail 2020;8(7):537–47.
9. Metra M, Cotter G, Senger S, et al. Prognostic Significance of Creatinine Increases During an Acute Heart Failure Admission in Patients With and Without Residual Congestion: A Post Hoc Analysis of the PROTECT Data. Circ Heart Fail 2018;11(5):e004644.
10. Hanberg JS, Sury K, Wilson FP, et al. Reduced Cardiac Index Is Not the Dominant Driver of Renal Dysfunction in Heart Failure. J Am Coll Cardiol 2016;67(19): 2199–208.
11. Nohria A, Hasselblad V, Stebbins A, et al. Cardiorenal interactions: insights from the ESCAPE trial. J Am Coll Cardiol 2008;51(13):1268–74.
12. Cuffe MS, Califf RM, Adams KF, et al. Short-term intravenous milrinone for acute exacerbation of chronic heart failure: a randomized controlled trial. JAMA 2002; 287(12):1541–7.
13. Klein L, Massie BM, Leimberger JD, et al. Admission or changes in renal function during hospitalization for worsening heart failure predict postdischarge survival: results from the Outcomes of a Prospective Trial of Intravenous Milrinone for Exacerbations of Chronic Heart Failure (OPTIME-CHF). Circ Heart Fail 2008;1(1): 25–33.
14. Teerlink JR, Diaz R, Felker GM, et al. Omecamtiv Mecarbil in Chronic Heart Failure With Reduced Ejection Fraction: Rationale and Design of GALACTIC-HF. JACC Heart Fail 2020;8(4):329–40.

15. Mullens W, Abrahams Z, Francis GS, et al. Importance of venous congestion for worsening of renal function in advanced decompensated heart failure. J Am Coll Cardiol 2009;53(7):589–96.

16. Testani JM, McCauley BD, Chen J, et al. Clinical characteristics and outcomes of patients with improvement in renal function during the treatment of decompensated heart failure. J Card Fail 2011;17(12):993–1000.

17. Dupont M, Mullens W, Finucan M, et al. Determinants of dynamic changes in serum creatinine in acute decompensated heart failure: the importance of blood pressure reduction during treatment. Eur J Heart Fail 2013;15(4):433–40.

18. McCallum W, Tighiouart H, Testani JM, et al. Association of Volume Overload With Kidney Function Outcomes Among Patients With Heart Failure With Reduced Ejection Fraction. Kidney Int Rep 2020;5(10):1661–9.

19. Burnett JC, Knox FG. Renal interstitial pressure and sodium excretion during renal vein constriction. Am J Physiol 1980;238(4):F279–82.

20. Hanberg JS, Rao V, Ter Maaten JM, et al. Hypochloremia and Diuretic Resistance in Heart Failure: Mechanistic Insights. Circ Heart Fail 2016;9(8). https://doi.org/ 10.1161/CIRCHEARTFAILURE.116.003180.

21. Mills RM, LeJemtel TH, Horton DP, et al. Sustained hemodynamic effects of an infusion of nesiritide (human b-type natriuretic peptide) in heart failure. J Am Coll Cardiol 1999;34(1):155–62.

22. Marcus LS, Hart D, Packer M, et al. Hemodynamic and renal excretory effects of human brain natriuretic peptide infusion in patients with congestive heart failure. A double-blind, placebo-controlled, randomized crossover trial. Circulation 1996; 94(12):3184–9.

23. O'Connor CM, Starling RC, Hernandez AF, et al. Effect of nesiritide in patients with acute decompensated heart failure. N Engl J Med 2011;365(1):32–43.

24. Chen HH, Anstrom KJ, Givertz MM, et al. Low-dose dopamine or low-dose nesiritide in acute heart failure with renal dysfunction: the ROSE acute heart failure randomized trial. JAMA 2013;310(23):2533–43.

25. Inker LA, Eneanya ND, Coresh J, et al. New Creatinine- and Cystatin C–Based Equations to Estimate GFR without Race. N Engl J Med 2021;385(19):1737–49.

26. Delgado C, Baweja M, Crews DC, et al. A Unifying Approach for GFR Estimation: Recommendations of the NKF-ASN Task Force on Reassessing the Inclusion of Race in Diagnosing Kidney Disease. J Am Soc Nephrol 2021;32(12):2994–3015.

27. Chen DC, Potok OA, Rifkin D, et al. Advantages, Limitations, and Clinical Considerations in Using Cystatin C to Estimate GFR. Kidney360 2022;3(10):1807.

28. Ahmad T, Jackson K, Rao VS, et al. Worsening Renal Function in Patients With Acute Heart Failure Undergoing Aggressive Diuresis Is Not Associated With Tubular Injury. Circulation 2018;137(19):2016–28.

29. Wettersten N, Horiuchi Y, van Veldhuisen DJ, et al. Short-term prognostic implications of serum and urine neutrophil gelatinase-associated lipocalin in acute heart failure: findings from the AKINESIS study. Eur J Heart Fail 2020;22(2):251–63.

30. Koyama S, Sato Y, Tanada Y, et al. Early evolution and correlates of urine albumin excretion in patients presenting with acutely decompensated heart failure. Circ Heart Fail 2013;6(2):227–32.

31. Mullens W, Damman K, Harjola VP, et al. The use of diuretics in heart failure with congestion - a position statement from the Heart Failure Association of the European Society of Cardiology. Eur J Heart Fail 2019;21(2):137–55.

32. Moghazi S, Jones E, Schroepple J, et al. Correlation of renal histopathology with sonographic findings. Kidney Int 2005;67(4):1515–20.

33. Beaubien-Souligny W, Benkreira A, Robillard P, et al. Alterations in Portal Vein Flow and Intrarenal Venous Flow Are Associated With Acute Kidney Injury After Cardiac Surgery: A Prospective Observational Cohort Study. J Am Heart Assoc 2018;7(19):e009961.
34. Iida N, Seo Y, Sai S, et al. Clinical Implications of Intrarenal Hemodynamic Evaluation by Doppler Ultrasonography in Heart Failure. JACC Heart Fail 2016;4(8): 674–82.
35. Lund LH, Benson L, Dahlström U, et al. Association Between Use of Renin-Angiotensin System Antagonists and Mortality in Patients With Heart Failure and Preserved Ejection Fraction. JAMA 2012;308(20):2108–17.
36. Yusuf S, Pfeffer MA, Swedberg K, et al. Effects of candesartan in patients with chronic heart failure and preserved left-ventricular ejection fraction: the CHARM-Preserved Trial. Lancet 2003;362(9386):777–81.
37. Massie BM, Carson PE, McMurray JJ, et al. Irbesartan in Patients with Heart Failure and Preserved Ejection Fraction. N Engl J Med 2008;359(23):2456–67.
38. Testani JM, Kimmel SE, Dries DL, et al. Prognostic importance of early worsening renal function after initiation of angiotensin-converting enzyme inhibitor therapy in patients with cardiac dysfunction. Circ Heart Fail 2011;4(6):685–91.
39. McCallum W, Tighiouart H, Ku E, et al. Acute declines in estimated glomerular filtration rate on enalapril and mortality and cardiovascular outcomes in patients with heart failure with reduced ejection fraction. Kidney Int 2019;96(5):1185–94.
40. McMurray JJV, Packer M, Desai AS, et al. Angiotensin–Neprilysin Inhibition versus Enalapril in Heart Failure. N Engl J Med 2014;371(11):993–1004.
41. Damman K, Gori M, Claggett B, et al. Renal Effects and Associated Outcomes During Angiotensin-Neprilysin Inhibition in Heart Failure. JACC Heart Fail 2018; 6(6):489–98.
42. Heidenreich PA, Bozkurt B, Aguilar D, et al. 2022 AHA/ACC/HFSA Guideline for the Management of Heart Failure: A Report of the American College of Cardiology/American Heart Association Joint Committee on Clinical Practice Guidelines. Circulation 2022;145(18):e895–1032.
43. Solomon SD, McMurray JJV, Anand IS, et al. Angiotensin-Neprilysin Inhibition in Heart Failure with Preserved Ejection Fraction. N Engl J Med 2019;381(17): 1609–20.
44. Mc Causland FR, Lefkowitz MP, Claggett B, et al. Angiotensin-Neprilysin Inhibition and Renal Outcomes in Heart Failure With Preserved Ejection Fraction. Circulation 2020;142(13):1236–45.
45. Mc Causland FR, Lefkowitz MP, Claggett B, et al. Angiotensin-neprilysin inhibition and renal outcomes across the spectrum of ejection fraction in heart failure. Eur J Heart Fail 2022;24(9):1591–8.
46. Remuzzi G, Cattaneo D, Perico N. The Aggravating Mechanisms of Aldosterone on Kidney Fibrosis: Figure 1. JASN (J Am Soc Nephrol) 2008;19(8):1459–62.
47. Edelmann F, Wachter R, Schmidt AG, et al. Effect of Spironolactone on Diastolic Function and Exercise Capacity in Patients With Heart Failure With Preserved Ejection Fraction: The Aldo-DHF Randomized Controlled Trial. JAMA 2013; 309(8):781–91.
48. Pitt B, Pfeffer MA, Assmann SF, et al. Spironolactone for Heart Failure with Preserved Ejection Fraction. N Engl J Med 2014;370(15):1383–92.
49. Butler J, Anker SD, Lund LH, et al. Patiromer for the management of hyperkalemia in heart failure with reduced ejection fraction: the DIAMOND trial. Eur Heart J 2022;ehac401. https://doi.org/10.1093/eurheartj/ehac401.

50. McDonagh TA, Metra M, Adamo M, et al. 2021 ESC Guidelines for the diagnosis and treatment of acute and chronic heart failure: Developed by the Task Force for the diagnosis and treatment of acute and chronic heart failure of the European Society of Cardiology (ESC) With the special contribution of the Heart Failure Association (HFA) of the ESC. Eur Heart J 2021;42(36):3599–726.

51. Rossing P, Caramori ML, Chan JCN, et al. Executive summary of the KDIGO 2022 Clinical Practice Guideline for Diabetes Management in Chronic Kidney Disease: an update based on rapidly emerging new evidence. Kidney Int 2022;102(5): 990–9.

52. Rovin BH, Adler SG, Barratt J, et al. Executive summary of the KDIGO 2021 Guideline for the Management of Glomerular Diseases. Kidney Int 2021;100(4): 753–79.

53. Anker SD, Butler J, Filippatos G, et al. Empagliflozin in Heart Failure with a Preserved Ejection Fraction. N Engl J Med 2021;385(16):1451–61.

54. Agarwal MA, Fonarow GC, Ziaeian B. National Trends in Heart Failure Hospitalizations and Readmissions From 2010 to 2017. JAMA Cardiol 2021;6(8):952–6.

55. Felker GM, Lee KL, Bull DA, et al. Diuretic strategies in patients with acute decompensated heart failure. N Engl J Med 2011;364(9):797–805.

56. Abdallah JG, Schrier RW, Edelstein C, et al. Loop diuretic infusion increases thiazide-sensitive Na(+)/Cl(-)-cotransporter abundance: role of aldosterone. J Am Soc Nephrol 2001;12(7):1335–41.

57. Trullàs JC, Morales-Rull JL, Casado J, et al. Combining loop with thiazide diuretics for decompensated heart failure: the CLOROTIC trial. Eur Heart J 2022;ehac689. https://doi.org/10.1093/eurheartj/ehac689.

58. Agarwal R, Sinha AD. Thiazide diuretics in advanced chronic kidney disease. J Am Soc Hypertens 2012;6(5):299–308.

59. Butler J, Anstrom KJ, Felker GM, et al. Efficacy and Safety of Spironolactone in Acute Heart Failure: The ATHENA-HF Randomized Clinical Trial. JAMA Cardiol 2017;2(9):950–8.

60. Mullens W, Dauw J, Martens P, et al. Acetazolamide in Acute Decompensated Heart Failure with Volume Overload. N Engl J Med 2022. https://doi.org/10. 1056/NEJMoa2203094.

61. Konstam MA, Gheorghiade M, Burnett JC, et al. Effects of oral tolvaptan in patients hospitalized for worsening heart failure: the EVEREST Outcome Trial. JAMA 2007;297(12):1319–31.

62. Hauptman PJ, Burnett J, Gheorghiade M, et al. Clinical course of patients with hyponatremia and decompensated systolic heart failure and the effect of vasopressin receptor antagonism with tolvaptan. J Card Fail 2013;19(6):390–7.

63. Costanzo MR, Guglin ME, Saltzberg MT, et al. Ultrafiltration versus intravenous diuretics for patients hospitalized for acute decompensated heart failure. J Am Coll Cardiol 2007;49(6):675–83.

64. Bart BA, Goldsmith SR, Lee KL, et al. Ultrafiltration in decompensated heart failure with cardiorenal syndrome. N Engl J Med 2012;367(24):2296–304.

65. Costanzo MR, Negoianu D, Jaski BE, et al. Aquapheresis Versus Intravenous Diuretics and Hospitalizations for Heart Failure. JACC Heart Fail 2016;4(2):95–105.

66. Greene SJ, Butler J, Albert NM, et al. Medical Therapy for Heart Failure With Reduced Ejection Fraction. J Am Coll Cardiol 2018;72(4):351–66.

67. Voors AA, Angermann CE, Teerlink JR, et al. The SGLT2 inhibitor empagliflozin in patients hospitalized for acute heart failure: a multinational randomized trial. Nat Med 2022;28(3):568–74.

68. Velazquez EJ, Morrow DA, DeVore AD, et al. Angiotensin–Neprilysin Inhibition in Acute Decompensated Heart Failure. N Engl J Med 2019;380(6):539–48.

69. Investigators SOLVD, Yusuf S, Pitt B, et al. Effect of enalapril on survival in patients with reduced left ventricular ejection fractions and congestive heart failure. N Engl J Med 1991;325(5):293–302.

70. McCallum W, Tighiouart H, Ku E, et al. Trends in Kidney Function Outcomes Following RAAS Inhibition in Patients With Heart Failure With Reduced Ejection Fraction. Am J Kidney Dis 2019. https://doi.org/10.1053/j.ajkd.2019.05.010.

71. Investigators SOLVD, Yusuf S, Pitt B, et al. Effect of enalapril on mortality and the development of heart failure in asymptomatic patients with reduced left ventricular ejection fractions. N Engl J Med 1992;327(10):685–91.

72. Zannad F, McMurray JJV, Krum H, et al. Eplerenone in Patients with Systolic Heart Failure and Mild Symptoms. N Engl J Med 2011;364(1):11–21.

73. Rossignol P, Dobre D, McMurray JJV, et al. Incidence, Determinants, and Prognostic Significance of Hyperkalemia and Worsening Renal Function in Patients With Heart Failure Receiving the Mineralocorticoid Receptor Antagonist Eplerenone or Placebo in Addition to Optimal Medical Therapy. Circulation: Heart Fail 2014;7(1):51–8.

74. Pitt B, Remme W, Zannad F, et al. Eplerenone, a selective aldosterone blocker, in patients with left ventricular dysfunction after myocardial infarction. N Engl J Med 2003;348(14):1309–21.

75. McMurray JJV, Solomon SD, Inzucchi SE, et al. Dapagliflozin in Patients with Heart Failure and Reduced Ejection Fraction. N Engl J Med 2019;381(21): 1995–2008.

76. Packer M, Anker SD, Butler J, et al. Cardiovascular and Renal Outcomes with Empagliflozin in Heart Failure. N Engl J Med 2020;383(15):1413–24.

Hepatorenal Syndrome
Pathophysiology, Diagnosis, and Treatment

Justin M. Belcher, MD, PhD

KEYWORDS

- Hepatorenal syndrome • Cirrhosis • Acute kidney injury (AKI) • Terlipressin
- Fractional excretion of sodium (FENa)

KEY POINTS

- Hepatorenal syndrome (HRS) is a primarily functional form of acute kidney injury that develops in patients with decompensated cirrhosis.
- The diagnosis of HRS is challenging and formal diagnostic criteria cannot always distinguish between patients with HRS and acute tubular necrosis.
- Objective tests including kidney biomarkers and the fractional excretion of sodium may allow for more accurate diagnosis.
- The standard of care for HRS is a combination of vasoconstrictor therapy and intravenous albumin.
- Terlipressin, a vasopressin analog, was recently approved for use in the United States and will likely be the first-line agent for treatment of HRS.

INTRODUCTION

Hospitalized patients with cirrhosis are at high risk for acute kidney injury (AKI), with rates ranging from 20% to 30% overall[1,2] and to more than 50% in patients admitted to intensive care units (ICUs).[2] AKI in this setting is increasingly common and this increase mirrors an overall increase in cirrhosis-associated admissions.[3,4] AKI is associated with significant morbidity and mortality, with in-hospital and 3-month mortality rates of 35% and 47%.[2,5] The most common causes of AKI in patients with cirrhosis are prerenal azotemia (PRA), acute tubular necrosis (ATN), and hepatorenal syndrome (HRS). This list is not comprehensive, however, and other causes including glomerulonephritis and acute interstitial nephritis may be present. Patients with AKI and cirrhosis are incredibly complex and these causes may overlap, with additional potential insults including abdominal compartment syndrome, cirrhotic cardiomyopathy, and bile-acid associated acute tubular injury further muddying the clinical picture. HRS, which constitutes between 15% and 30% of AKI in this setting,[5,6] has long been one of the most

Section of Nephrology, Yale University School of Medicine, VA Connecticut Healthcare System, VA Connecticut Healthcare, Room G126B, 950 Campbell Avenue, West Haven, CT 06516, USA
E-mail address: Justin.belcher@yale.edu
Twitter: @jmbnephdoc (J.M.B.)

Med Clin N Am 107 (2023) 781–792
https://doi.org/10.1016/j.mcna.2023.03.009
0025-7125/23/Published by Elsevier Inc.

medical.theclinics.com

feared complications of advanced cirrhosis and is associated with a 90-day mortality rate of 50% to 80%.[7] HRS has classically been subdivided as Type 1, which occurs rapidly after a precipitating event and is nearly universally fatal if untreated, and Type 2, which is more indolent and associated with refractory ascites. Recent updates in diagnostic criteria and nomenclature have renamed HRS-1, which will be the subject of this review, as HRS-AKI.[8] Distinguishing patients with HRS-AKI from those with other AKI causes is critical because treatment strategies vary widely. However, making this diagnostic distinction presents a formidable clinical challenge because diagnostic criteria are often nonspecific, and patients may have pathophysiologic features of more than one condition. Along with updated diagnostic criteria, newly available treatment options and diagnostic tests present the hope of improved outcomes in these critically ill patients. This review will summarize the pathophysiology, diagnostic approach to and treatment options for patients with HRS-AKI.

PATHOPHYSIOLOGY

HRS-AKI has historically been conceptualized as a purely functional form of renal failure, where glomerular filtration rate fell due to renal hypoperfusion rather than frank structural injury. This model was supported by experimental studies demonstrating that failed kidneys from patients deceased with HRS resumed function when transplanted into recipients without cirrhosis.[9] Biopsies of kidneys from patients with HRS have typically demonstrated very less histologic damage, even under electron microscopy.[10] The pathologic cascade resulting in HRS-AKI begins in the setting of cirrhosis with liver fibrosis and regenerative nodules.[11,12] This leads to an increased intrahepatic vascular resistance and sinusoidal/portal hypertension and subsequently to an overexpression of compensatory vasodilatory substances. The accumulation of such vasodilatory factors, including nitric oxide and endogenous cannabinoids, leads to a hyperdynamic splanchnic circulatory state and increased shear stress, which along with increased intestinal permeability related to portal hypertension, results in bacterial translocation, further augmenting vasodilatation. As a result, blood is sequestered in the splanchnic vascular bed leading to diminished effective circulating arterial blood volume[11] and a reduction in systemic vascular resistance and mean arterial pressure (MAP). These physiologic changes are depicted in **Fig. 1**.

Initially, increases in cardiac contractility and cardiac output counterbalance the reduction in systemic vascular resistance to maintain end-organ perfusion. Achieving this increase, however, requires depletion of cardiac functional reserves as demonstrated by Koshy and colleagues.[13] In this study, 560 patients undergoing workup for liver transplantation received a dobutamine stress echocardiogram. Of these, 64 (13%) had established HRS. These patients with HRS had a significantly higher baseline cardiac output but a blunted response to dobutamine. Of those without HRS, 94 (22%) developed it during a median of 1.5 years follow-up. A significantly higher proportion of those with low cardiac reserved, defined as a less than 25% increase in cardiac output with dobutamine, developed HRS 52 (55%) versus 56 (17%). Eventually, even baseline cardiac output begins to fall due to the development of cirrhotic cardiomyopathy. In response, compensatory neurohormonal vasoconstrictor systems such as the renin-angiotensin-aldosterone system (RAAS), the sympathetic nervous system (SNS), and arginine vasopressin are stimulated to augment intravascular volume and blood pressure and defend end-organ perfusion. The cumulative effect of activating these systems is increased renal sodium and water retention, worsening existing ascites and hyponatremia, and progressive renal vasoconstriction. Secondary hits, including spontaneous bacterial peritonitis, acute on chronic liver failure (ACLF),

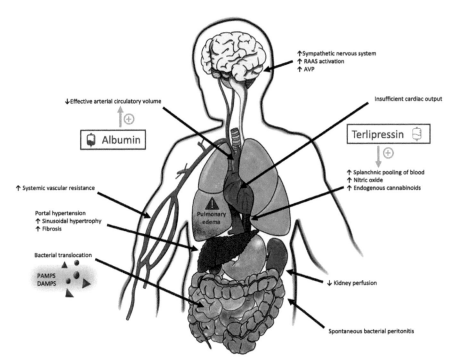

Fig. 1. Physiologic derangements leading to hepatorenal syndrome and effects of terlipressin. Depicted are the organ systems and physiologic derangements involved in the development of hepatorenal syndrome. Albumin exerts its primary effect by increasing intravascular oncotic pressure and preventing third spacing of fluids. Vasoconstrictors (here represented by terlipressin) act to constrict the splanchnic system, shunting blood back to systemic circulation, and increasing effective circulating volume. The resulting reduced activation of the sympathetic nervous system, renin-angiotensin-aldosterone axis, and release of arginine vasopressin ameliorates renal vascular vasoconstriction and improves renal perfusion. AVP, arginine vasopressin; DAMPs, pathogen-associated molecular patterns; PAMPs, damage-associated molecular patterns; RAAS, renin-angiotensin-aldosterone system. (Justin M. Belcher et al., Terlipressin and the Treatment of Hepatorenal Syndrome: How the CONFIRM Trial Moves the Story Forward, American Journal of Kidney Diseases, 79 (5), 2022, 737-745, https://doi.org/10.1053/j.ajkd.2021.08.016. Courtesy of the National Kidney Foundation.)

variceal bleeding, or even excessive use of diuretics or lactulose may further potentiate intrarenal vasoconstriction, ultimately overwhelming local vasodilators, and resulting in a severe decline in renal blood flow, reduced GFR, and the rapidly progressive, volume-unresponsive renal failure that characterizes HRS-AKI.[14]

Although this standard conceptualization of the pathophysiology of HRS-AKI is indeed accurate, it has more recently become increasingly apparent that it is incomplete. Evidence of systemic inflammation has been found in up to one-third of patients with HRS-AKI who lack any evidence of documented infection.[15] Such inflammation may be due to sterile inflammatory processes such as alcoholic hepatitis or acute-on-chronic liver failure or translocation of bacterial lipopolysaccharides. The resulting release of damage-associated molecular pathways and pathogen-associated molecular pathways, respectively, triggers further production of inflammatory and vasoactive cytokines and chemokines.[16] These molecules may potentiate the severity of AKI via direct injury to renal tubules mediated by the formation of microthrombi in the renal microvasculature[17–19] and by driving further RAAS and SNS activation.

DIAGNOSIS
Standard Criteria

With no specific histologic findings or serologic markers and often triggered by precipitating factors capable of inducing alternative etiologies of AKI (PRA, ATN), the diagnosis of HRS has historically been one of exclusion. To assist clinicians in parsing this challenging distinction, multiple sets of diagnostic criteria have been proposed. Based on the conception of HRS as a purely functional and volume refractory form of AKI, HRS diagnostic criteria, primarily developed by the International Ascites Club (IAC), have sought to identify patients with HRS by excluding those with evidence of PRA or ATN. The most recent set of IAC criteria was published in 2015 and is presented in **Box 1**.[20] The most critical update was the elimination of any specific creatinine threshold for the diagnosis of HRS. Earlier versions had mandated a creatinine value of at least 1.5 mg/dL and, for the diagnosis of HRS-1, a value of at least 2.5 mg/dL with either a doubling of creatinine or halving of glomerular filtration rate during 2 weeks. However, due to decreased creatine synthesis, loss of muscle mass, poor protein intake, and increased volume of distribution, patients with advanced cirrhosis frequently have a low baseline creatinine level. The requirement therefore of an absolute creatinine threshold before the diagnosis of HRS could be made likely delayed the initiation of therapy and reduced the likelihood of response. The current criteria have abolished a threshold and only require patients to meet the standard Kidney Disease: Improving Global Outcomes (KDIGO) AKI definition of an increase in creatinine of at least 0.3 mg/dL from baseline during 48 hours or a 50% increase during 7 days.[21]

Biomarkers

Although adequate volume expansion should identify patients with PRA, parsing those with HRS-AKI from ATN often remains clinically challenging and a definitive diagnosis may be elusive. Novel biomarkers released only in the setting of overt tubular injury demonstrate the ability to distinguish functional from structural AKI in multiple settings[22] and hold great promise in patients with cirrhosis. Acknowledging this, the 2015 iteration of the IAC criteria noted that patients may fulfill all 5 criteria yet still

---

Box 1
International Ascites Club Diagnostic Criteria for HRS-AKI

Diagnostic Criteria for HRS-AKI

Diagnosis of cirrhosis and ascites

Diagnosis of AKI according to AKI-IAC criteria[a]

No response after 2 consecutive days of diuretic withdrawal and plasma volume expansion with albumin at 1 g/kg of bodyweight

Absence of shock

No current or recent use of nephrotoxic drugs

No macroscopic signs of structural kidney injury, defines as:
- Absence of proteinuria (>500 mg/d)
- Absence of microscopic hematur0a (>50 RBCs per high power field)
- Normal findings on renal ultrasound

[a]AKI-IAC definition of AKI is taken from that of Kidney Disease: Improving Global Outcomes (KDIGO) definition.[21]*Abbreviations:* AKI, acute kidney injury; HRS, hepatorenal syndrome; RBC, red blood cell.

have tubular injury and highlighted the potential of biomarkers to assist with diagnostic distinctions.[20] Multiple candidate biomarkers have been investigated but the most extensively studied has been neutrophil gelatinase-associated lipocalin (NGAL).[23] Across multiple studies, NGAL has demonstrated a stepwise increase across diagnoses from PRA to HRS to ATN.[24–27] NGAL values for the 3 diagnoses reflecting the marked consistency across adjudicated studies are shown in **Fig. 2**. Although an optimal cut point has not been formally established, a value adjusted for urinary creatinine of ~220 to 250 µg/g is consistent with much of the data.

In identifying patients as having HRS, biomarkers may be able to predict which patients will respond to HRS-specific therapy, thereby limiting exposure to potential medication side effects in patients unlikely to receive any benefit from treatment. Critically, a recent study by Gambino and colleagues[31] tested the hypothesis that urinary NGAL levels can predict the response to modern HRS-AKI therapy. One hundred sixty-two consecutive patients with cirrhosis and AKI were enrolled including 35 (22%) with PRA, 64 (40%) with HRS-AKI, 27 (17%) with ATN and 36 (22%) with "mixed" (unadjudicable) AKI. Mean NGAL was significantly higher in ATN than in other types of AKI ([1162 ng/mL (423–2105 ng/mL)] verses [109 ng/mL (52–192 ng/mL)]; $P < .001$). NGAL had a strong ability to discrimination ATN (AUC 0.854 [95% CI 0.767–0.941], $P < .001$) with an optimal cutoff of 220 ng/mL. Sixty-four patients were diagnosed with HRS and treated with terlipressin (see later discussion). Of these, 38 (59%) patients responded to treatment. Patients with NGAL less than 220 ng/mL were significantly more likely to respond, 70% versus 33%, $P = .015$. It is possible a panel of injury markers may perform better than any single candidate.[25]

Despite these encouraging data, there remains an overlap in the distribution of values for NGAL and other biomarkers between patients with HRS-AKI and ATN. This is to be expected because patients exist on a spectrum of functional to structural

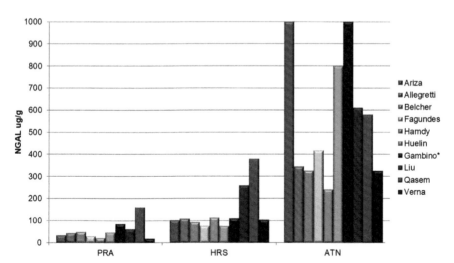

Fig. 2. NGAL values across diagnoses of AKI in patients with cirrhosis. NGAL values for patients diagnosed with PRA, HRS, and ATN across studies. In each study, the difference between values for HRS and ATN is statistically significant. Values for Ariza and Gambino were winsorized at 1000 µg/g for clarity of depiction. *, Gambino is reported in nanograms per milliliter, not microgram per gram.[24–33] NGAL, neutrophil gelatinase-associated lipocalin; PRA, pre-renal azotemia.

disease. What is really needed is not a means of determining which condition the patient "has" but rather a means of prospectively identifying which patients' AKI is likely to resolve with restoration of renal perfusion. To infer this, it is necessary to assess not only the degree of tubular injury but also residual tubular functional integrity. The fractional excretion of sodium (FENa) is a mainstay of nephrologists in attempts to distinguish functional (PRA) from structural (ATN) AKI but has often been considered unhelpful in patients with advanced liver disease.[34] Such patients manifest near universal sodium avidity such that FENa is virtually always less than the traditional diagnostic cutoff of 1%, even in those without AKI and, at times, even in those with ATN. However, multiple studies have shown FENa can indeed reliably distinguish ATN from HRS-AKI in adjudicated patients when cutoffs are reconsidered, with values for HRS-AKI patients typically less than 0.2% and often less than 0.1%. FENa values for PRA, HRS-AKI, and ATN across studies are shown in **Fig. 3**. It is possible that the IAC criteria may be amended to include an FENa value less than 0.2%.[8]

Many patients with advanced cirrhosis and ascites are on diuretics before the onset of AKI, and their use can complicate the interpretation of FENa. Few studies have assessed the performance of the fractional excretion of urea (FEUrea) as an alternative to FENa. Patidar and colleagues,[37] in a study of 50 patients with cirrhosis and AKI, found an AUC of 0.96, with an optimal cutoff of 33.4%, for the ability of FEUrea to distinguish ATN versus non-ATN, 0.87 (cutoff 28.7%) to identify HRS versus non-HRS, and 0.81 (cutoff 21.6% for HRS versus PRA. FENa was not assessed in the study. In contrast, Gowda and colleagues[35] investigated both biomarkers in 200 patients and found FENa to significantly outperform FEUrea in discriminating both ATN versus non-ATN (AUC 87% vs 60%) and HRS versus non-HRS (AUC 75% vs 60%). Other markers of tubular functional integrity including urine cystatin C await further study.[25] Future biomarker panels attempting to accurately phenotype AKI in

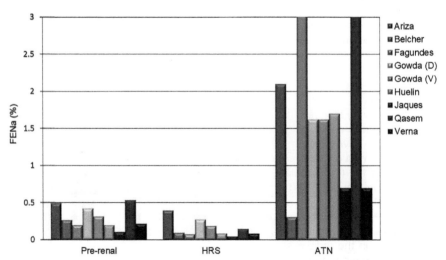

Fig. 3. FENa values across diagnoses of AKI in patients with cirrhosis. FENa values for patients diagnosed with PRA, HRS, and ATN across studies. In each study, the difference between values for PRA and HRS and between HRS and ATN were statistically significant. Values for Fagundes and Qasem were winsorized at 3% for clarity of depiction.[24,25,27–29,33,35,36] Gowda and colleagues included a derivation (D) and validation (V) cohort in their study, the results of each are depicted separately. AKI, acute kidney injury; PRA, pre-renal azotemia.

patients with cirrhosis may also include markers assessing the intensity of systemic vasodilatation and renal vasoconstriction.[32]

TREATMENT
Vasopressors

The ultimate treatment of HRS-AKI is liver transplantation, which reverses the physiology leading to renal hypoperfusion. When this is not possible, the foundational therapy for HRS consists of vasoconstrictor therapy paired with volume expansion in the form of albumin. By inducing vasoconstriction of the splanchnic system, blood is shunted to the systemic system, increasing MAP and effective circulating arterial volume, thereby reducing activation of the RAAS and CNS, reducing renal vasoconstriction, and restoring renal perfusion. If approved alternatives are not available, the off-label use of midodrine (an oral α-receptor agonist prodrug) and somatostatin (an octreotide analog serving to decrease the production of splanchnic vasodilatory substances) has been the most utilized vasoconstrictor therapy in the United States.

Despite widespread use, there are limited data supporting the efficacy of the midodrine/octreotide combination.[38] Evidence of benefit has been confined to uncontrolled retrospective cohort studies.[39] In one of the few randomized comparative trials, HRS-AKI patients treated with terlipressin had a significantly higher rate of renal recovery (70%) compared with midodrine/octreotide (29%).[40,41] When, as frequently occurs, midodrine/octreotide is ineffective, patients in the United States are often treated with norepinephrine. Although norepinephrine has been clearly demonstrated to be superior to midodrine/octreotide,[41] its administration typically requires admission to an ICU and placement of a central venous line, generally rendering it a second-line therapy. In much of the world, including Europe, Asia, and parts of Latin America, the first-line treatment of HRS-AKI is terlipressin,[42] paired with albumin. Terlipressin is a vasopressin analog with a greater affinity for the V1 receptor than vasopressin, a more prolonged course of action and greater affinity for the splanchnic vasculature bed.[43,44] Critically, it can be given through peripheral access and on a regular medical floor, saving the cost of ICU admissions and the hazards of central access placement. Following 2 trials, OT-0401[45] and REVERSE,[46] with borderline positive findings, terlipressin was recently approved for use in the Unites States based on results of the CONFIRM trial.[47] Eligible patients were required to have creatinine of 2.25 mg/dL or greater and were randomized 2:1 with 199 receiving terlipressin and 101, placebo. The primary endpoint was defined as a fall in creatinine to 1.5 mg/dL or lesser on 2 consecutive measurements while on treatment and alive and dialysis-free 10 days after the second value. The trial achieved this, with 63 out of 199 (32%) patients in the terlipressin arm as compared with 17 out of 101 (17%) patients in the placebo arm reaching the primary endpoint, $P = .006$. The trial examined 4 prespecified secondary end points. Three of them, HRS reversal (defined as at least one creatinine value while on treatment less than 1.5 mg/dL), HRS reversal with no renal-replacement therapy through 30 days, and HRS reversal in patients with systemic inflammatory response syndrome were significantly higher in the terlipressin arm. The fourth secondary endpoint, Verified HRS reversal with no recurrence through 30 days favored terlipressin but did not meet statistical significance. Importantly, terlipressin-treated subjects had a greater incidence of respiratory adverse events. It is possible that aggressive administration of intravenous albumin both before enrollment and while on protocol may have played a role in the increased incidence of respiratory failure and fluid overload. Subgroup analysis identified patients with creatinine 5 mg/dL or greater and those with ACLF Grade 3 as being at particular risk of respiratory events and terlipressin should only be used with significant caution in such cases.

Several small trials have compared norepinephrine and terlipressin and found generally comparable outcomes.[48,49] In the largest and most recent trial, Arora and colleagues[50] randomized 120 patients with HRS-AKI (all of whom had ACLF) to either continuous infusion of terlipressin or norepinephrine, both accompanied by albumin. Patients treated with terlipressin had significantly greater rates of HRS reversal (40% vs 17%, P = .03) and 28-day survival (48% vs 20%, P = .001) and significantly lower requirement for the renal replacement therapy (RRT; 57% vs 80%, P = .006). Importantly, patients treated with terlipressin had significantly higher rates of adverse events related to use of the drug, 23% versus 8%, P = .02, although there was no difference in respiratory events.

Transjugular Intrahepatic Portosystemic Shunt

Placement of a transjugular intrahepatic portosystemic shunt (TIPS) reduces portal pressure and is used in patients with portal hypertension suffering from refractory ascites or variceal bleeding. In theory, TIPS should be an effective means of treating HRS by shunting blood back to the systemic circulation (although with the associated risk of worsening hepatic encephalopathy), thereby reducing the stimulus for RAAS and SNS activation. Unfortunately, few studies have investigated this supposition. A meta-analysis included 9 study totaling 128 patients (77 with HRS-1 and 55 with HRS-2) found significant improvements in creatinine, serum sodium and urine output in both groups.[51] However, in only 2 studies was TIPS used following vasoconstrictor therapy, and it remains to be determined if and where in an HRS treatment algorithm TIPS should be considered. At present then TIPS should only be considered as a possible salvage therapy.

Renal Replacement Therapy

The role of RRT in patients with HRS has historically be controversial, both medically and ethically, as to whether it can be done and, separately, whether it should be done. Never risk free, the use of RRT in patients with cirrhosis is especially fraught with potential complications including intradialytic hypotension and hemodynamic instability, infection and the bleeding risks inherent in placing intravenous access in often thrombocytopenic and coagulopathic patients. Continuous RRT is often preferred over intermittent to mitigate some of these risks but carries its own challenges regarding anticoagulation. The timing of the initiation of RRT often adds to the challenges. Patients considered for dialysis have generally failed pharmacologic therapy and are thus often in extremis from volume overload and/or metabolic and electrolyte disturbances. Even if these challenges can be surmounted, many practitioners struggle as to whether RRT is ethically appropriate to pursue in patients with HRS-AKI. Dialysis does not address the underlying pathologic condition of end-stage cirrhosis. Instead, it has traditionally been thought of as a bridge in patients who are transplant eligible to sustain them until graft availability. Its use may extend life expectancy for several weeks to a few months.[52] However, prolonged utilization of RRT pretransplant is associated with negative graft and renal outcomes posttransplant.[53] In patients not eligible for transplant, RRT has been associated with short-term mortality exceeding 90%.[54] Many practitioners have therefore considered listing status when deciding whether to offer RRT and withheld it as inappropriate and futile in noneligible patients. In making this decision, however, a distinction has often been made between patients with HRS and those with ATN where, even when ineligible for transplant, RRT has often been offered as a means of "riding out" the ATN until renal recovery. Although this approach again does not address the dominant underlying pathologic condition, ATN itself is not necessarily fatal and patients who are able to come off of dialysis have been thought to have the potential for prolonged survival. In the largest study to date, Allegretti and colleagues[55] examined 472 patients with cirrhosis and AKI initiated on RRT. Of those, 341 (72%) were not listed for liver transplant. Interestingly, for the 56 (16%) HRS and 285 (84%) ATN unlisted patients, there was no difference in survival time, 21 (inter-quartile range [IQR] 8–70) versus 12 (3–43) days, P = .25, and, in multivariable analysis, etiology of AKI had no impact on 6-month survival for either listed or unlisted patients. Depending on one's perspective on medical decision-making, resource utilization and aggression of care, these data could suggest that nonlisted patients with HRS all be offered RRT because they have the same projected outcomes as patients with ATN. Alternatively, one could argue instead that the patients with ATN not be offered RRT because they may fare no better than those with HRS. Attempting to determine if there was any utility pursuing long-term RRT in patients with HRS-AKI, McAllister and colleagues. utilized the United States Renal Data System to identify 7830 patients discharged from 1996 to 2015 on chronic, maintenance RRT with their end-stage renal disease coded as attributable to HRS.[56] Three hundred ninety-three (6%) Medicare patients received a liver transplant within 1 year of follow-up, with 216 (55%) being simultaneous liver kidney transplants. Overall, 3120 (40%) patients were alive at 1 year. Although this is certainly a nonrepresentative sample of patients with HRS started on acute RRT (selecting out only those who survived to discharge), it does suggest that if patients with more favorable, short-term prospects can be identified, initiation of RRT even in those not eligible for transplant may be reasonable. This remains an area of considerable controversy and requires further study.

CLINICS CARE POINTS

- Although not part of the official diagnostic criteria, patients who truly have HRS-AKI are virtually always hyponatremic and have urine sodium less than 20 mmol/L, with an FENa of less than 0.2%.

- Although treatment algorithms recommend daily IV albumin along with vasoconstrictor therapy, daily assessments of volume status should be performed and albumin held if patients are showing signs of respiratory compromise.

- All therapies for HRS-AKI become less effective the higher the serum creatinine is at the initiation of treatment. Patients should be rapidly appraised when there is suspicion for HRS-AKI and definitive therapy started as quickly as possible.

DISCLOSURE

Dr J.M. Belcher has served on an advisory board for Mallinckrodt Pharmaceuticals, manufacturer of terlipressin.

REFERENCES

1. Hampel H, Bynum GD, Zamora E, et al. Risk factors for the development of renal dysfunction in hospitalized patients with cirrhosis. Am J Gastroenterol 2001;96: 2206–10.
2. Tariq R, Hadi Y, Chahal K, et al. Incidence, mortality and predictors of acute kidney injury in patients with cirrhosis: a systematic review and meta-analysis. J Clin Transl Hepatol 2020;8(2):135–42.

3. Desai AP, Knapp SM, Orman ES, et al. Changing epidemiology and outcomes of acute kidney injury in hospitalized patients with cirrhosis - a US population-based study. J Hepatol 2020;73(5):1092–9.
4. Pant C, Jani BS, Desai M, et al. Hepatorenal syndrome in hospitalized patients with chronic liver disease: results from the Nationwide Inpatient Sample 2002-2012. J Investig Med 2016;64(1):33–8.
5. Allegretti AS, Ortiz G, Wenger J, et al. Prognosis of acute kidney injury and hepatorenal syndrome in patients with cirrhosis: a prospective cohort study. Int J Hepatol 2015;108139. https://doi.org/10.1155/2015/108139.
6. Garcia-Tsao G, Parikh CR, Viola A. Acute kidney injury in cirrhosis. Hepatology 2008;48(6):2064–77.
7. Belcher JM, Parada XV, Simonetto DA, et al. Terlipressin and the treatment of hepatorenal syndrome: How the CONFIRM trial moves the story forward. Am J Kidney Dis 2022;79(5):737–45.
8. Angeli P, Garcia-Tsao G, Nadim MK, et al. New in the pathophysiology, definition and classification of hepatorenal syndrome: a step beyond the International Club of Ascites (ICA) consensus document. J Hepatol 2019;71(4):811–22.
9. Koppel MH, Coburn JW, Mims MM, et al. Transplantation of cadaveric kidneys from patients with hepatorenal syndrome- Evidence for the functional nature of renal failure in advanced liver disease. N Engl J Med 1969;280:1367–71.
10. Epstein M. Hepatorenal syndrome: emerging perspectives of pathophysiology and therapy. J Am Soc Nephrol 1994;4(10):1735–53.
11. Simonetto DA, Ginès P, Kamath PS. Hepatorenal syndrome: pathophysiology, diagnosis and management. BMJ 2020;370:m2687.
12. Ginès P, Solà E, Angeli P, et al. Hepatorenal syndrome. Nat Rev Dis Primers 2018; 4(1):23.
13. Koshy AN, Farouque O, Cailes B, et al. Impaired cardiac reserve on dobutamine stress echocardiography predicts the development of hepatorenal syndrome. Am J Gastroenterol 2020;115(3):388–97.
14. Velez JCQ, Therapondos G, Juncos LA. Reappraising the spectrum of AKI and hepatorenal syndrome in patients with cirrhosis. Nat Rev Nephrol 2020;16(3): 137–55.
15. Thabut D, Massard J, Gangloff A, et al. Model for end- stage liver disease score and systemic inflammatory response are major prognostic factors in patients with cirrhosis and acute functional renal failure. Hepatology 2007;46:1872–82.
16. Arroyo V, Angeli P, Moreau R, et al. The systemic inflammation hypothesis: towards a new paradigm of acute decompensation and multiorgan failure in cirrhosis. J Hepatol 2021;74:670–85.
17. Mihm S. Danger-associated molecular patterns (DAMPs): molecular triggers for sterile inflammation in the liver. Int J Mol Sci 2018;19(10):3104.
18. Fani F, Regolisti G, Delsante M, et al. Recent advances in the pathogenetic mechanisms of sepsis-associated acute kidney injury. J Nephrol 2018;31:351–9.
19. Earley LE. Presentation of diagnostic criteria of the hepatorenal syndrome. In: Bartoli E, Chiandussi L, editors. Hepatorenal syndrome. Padova: Piccin Medical Books; 1979. p. 495–504.
20. Angeli P, Ginès P, Wong F, et al. Diagnosis and management of acute kidney injury in patients with cirrhosis: revised consensus recommendations of the International Club of Ascites. Gut 2015;64(4):531–7.
21. Kellum JA, Lameire N, Aspelin P, et al. Kidney disease: improving global outcomes (KDIGO) acute kidney injury work group. KDIGO clinical practice guideline for acute kidney injury. Kidney Int 2012;2(Suppl 1):1–138.

22. Belcher JM, Edelstein CL, Parikh CR. Clinical applications of biomarkers for acute kidney injury. Am J Kidney Dis 2011;57(6):930–40.

23. Yewale RV, Ramakrishna BS. Novel biomarkers of acute kidney injury in chronic liver disease: where do we stand after a decade of research? Hepatol Res 2023;53(1):3–17.

24. Verna EC, Brown RS, Farrand E, et al. Urinary neutrophil gelatinase-associated lipocalin predicts mortality and identifies acute kidney injury in cirrhosis. Dig Dis Sci 2012;57:2362–70.

25. Belcher JM, Sanyal AJ, Peixoto AJ, et al. Kidney biomarkers and differential diagnosis of patients with cirrhosis and acute kidney injury. Hepatology 2014;60: 622–32.

26. Allegretti AS, Parada XV, Endres P, et al. Urinary NGAL as a diagnostic and prognostic marker for acute kidney injury in cirrhosis: A prospective study. Clin Transl Gastroenterol 2021;12(5):e00359.

27. Huelin P, Solà E, Elia C, et al. Neutrophil gelatinase-associated lipocalin for assessment of acute kidney injury in cirrhosis: A prospective study. Hepatology 2019;70(1):319–33.

28. Ariza X, Solà E, Elia C, et al. Analysis of a urinary biomarker panel for clinical outcomes assessment in cirrhosis. PLoS One 2015;10(6):e0128145.

29. Fagundes C, Pépin MN, Guevara M, et al. Urinary neutrophil gelatinase-associated lipocalin as biomarker in the differential diagnosis of impairment of kidney function in cirrhosis. J Hepatol 2012;57(2):267–73.

30. Hamdy HS, El-Ray A, Salaheldin M, et al. Urinary neutrophil gelatinase-associated lipocalin in cirrhotic patients with acute kidney injury. Ann Hepatol 2018;17(4):624–30.

31. Gambino C, Piano S, Stenico M, et al. Diagnostic and prognostic performance of urinary neutrophil gelatinase-associated lipocalin in patients with cirrhosis and acute kidney injury. Hepatology 2022. https://doi.org/10.1002/hep.32799.

32. Liu CW, Huang CC, Tsai HC, et al. Serum adrenomedullin and urinary thromboxane B_2 help early categorizing of acute kidney injury in decompensated cirrhotic patients: A prospective cohort study. Hepatol Res 2018;48(3):E9–21.

33. Qasem AA, Farag SE, Hamed E, et al. Urinary biomarkers of acute kidney injury in patients with cirrhosis. ISRN Nephrol 2014;2014:376795.

34. Diamond JR, Yoburn DC. Nonoligouric acute renal failure associated with a low fractional excretion of sodium. Ann Intern Med 1982;96:597–600.

35. Gowda YHS, Jagtap N, Karyampudi A, et al. Fractional excretion of sodium and urea in differentiating acute kidney injury phenotypes in decompensated cirrhosis. J Clin Exp Hepatol 2022;12(3):899–907.

36. Jaques DA, Spahr L, Berra G, et al. Biomarkers for acute kidney injury in decompensated cirrhosis: a prospective study. Nephrology 2019;24(2):170–80.

37. Patidar KR, Kang L, Bajaj JS, et al. Fractional excretion of urea: a simple tool for the differential diagnosis of acute kidney injury in cirrhosis. Hepatology 2018; 68(1):224–33.

38. Esrailian E, Pantangco ER, Kyulo NL, et al. Octreotide/midodrine therapy significantly improves renal function and 30-day survival in patients with type 1 hepatorenal syndrome. Dig Dis Sci 2007;52:742–8.

39. Skagen C, Einstein M, Lucey MR, et al. Combination treatment with octreotide, midodrine, and albumin improves survival in patients with Type 1 and Type 2 hepatorenal syndrome. J Clin Gastroenterol 2009;43:680–5.

40. Cavallin M, Kamath PS, Merli M, et al. Terlipressin plus albumin versus midodrine and octreotide plus albumin in the treatment of hepatorenal syndrome: A randomized trial. Hepatology 2015;62:567–74.

41. Mahmoud EIE, Abdelaziz DH, Abd-Elsalam S, et al. Norepinephrine is more effective than midodrine/octreotide in patients with hepatorenal syndrome-acute kidney injury: a randomized controlled trial. Front Pharmacol 2021;12: 675948.

42. EASL clinical practice guidelines for the management of patients with decompensated cirrhosis. J Hepatol 2018;69:406–60.

43. Jamil K, Pappas SC, Devarakonda KR. In vitro binding and receptor-mediated activity of terlipressin at vasopressin receptors V1 and V2. J Exp Pharmacol 2017;10:1–7.

44. Colson PH, Virsolvy A, Gaudard P, et al. Terlipressin, a vasoactive prodrug recommended in hepatorenal syndrome, is an agonist of human V1, V2 and V1B receptors: Implications for its safety profile. Pharmacol Res 2016;113(Pt A):257–64.

45. Sanyal AJ, Boyer T, Garcia-Tsao G, et al. A randomized, prospective, double-blind, placebo-controlled trial of terlipressin for type 1 hepatorenal syndrome. Gastroenterology 2008;134(5):1360–8.

46. Boyer T, Sanyal AJ, Wong F, et al. Terlipressin plus albumin is more effective than albumin alone in improving renal function in patients with cirrhosis and hepatorenal syndrome type 1. Gastroenterology 2016;150:1579–89.

47. Wong F, Pappas SC, Curry MP, et al. Terlipressin plus albumin for the treatment of type 1 hepatorenal syndrome. N Engl J Med 2021;384(9):818–28.

48. Badawy SSI, Meckawy NM, Ahmed A. Norepinephrine versus terlipressin in patients with type 1 hepatorenal syndrome refractory to treatment with octreotide, midodrine, and albumin: a prospective randomized comparative study. Egypt J Cardiothorac Anesth 2013;7:13–8.

49. Mattos ÂZ, Mattos AA, Ribeiro RA. Terlipressin versus noradrenaline in the treatment of hepatorenal syndrome: systematic review with meta-analysis and full economic evaluation. Eur J Gastroenterol Hepatol 2016;28(3):345–51.

50. Arora V, Maiwall R, Rajan V, et al. Terlipressin is superior to noradrenaline in the management of acute kidney injury in acute on chronic liver failure. Hepatology 2020;71(2):600–10.

51. Song T, Rössle M, He F, et al. Transjugular intrahepatic portosystemic shunt for hepatorenal syndrome- A systematic review and meta-analysis. Dig Liver Dis 2018;50(4):323–30.

52. Boyer TD, Sanyal AJ, Garcia-Tsao G, et al. Impact of liver transplantation on the survival of patients treated for hepatorenal syndrome type 1. Liver Transpl 2011; 17(11):1328–32.

53. Sharma P, Goodrich NP, Zhang M, et al. Short-term pretransplant renal replacement therapy and renal nonrecovery after liver transplantation. Clin J Am Soc Nephrol 2013;8(7):1135–42.

54. Wong LP, Blackley MP, Andreoni KA, et al. Survival of liver transplant candidates with acute renal failure receiving renal replacement therapy. Kidney Int 2005; 68(1):362–70.

55. Allegretti AS, Parada XV, Eneanya ND, et al. Prognosis of patients with cirrhosis and AKI who initiate RRT. Clin J Am Soc Nephrol 2018;13:16–25.

56. McAllister S, Lai JC, Copeland TP, et al. Renal recovery and mortality risk among patients with hepatorenal syndrome receiving chronic maintenance dialysis. Kidney360 2021;2(5):819–27.

Printed and bound by CPI Group (UK) Ltd, Croydon, CR0 4YY

03/10/2024

01040470-0013